AGING ISSUES, HEALTH AND FINANCIAL ALTERNATIVES

VETERANS BENEFITS: A SELECTION OF PROGRAMS FOR SERVICE MEMBERS

GEORGE B. MEYERS
AND
ALICE M. GLASKIN
EDITORS

Nova Science Publishers, Inc.
New York

For permission to use material from this book please contact us:
Telephone 631-231-7269; Fax 631-231-8175
Web Site: http://www.novapublishers.com

LIBRARY OF CONGRESS CATALOGING-IN-PUBLICATION DATA

Veterans benefits : a selection of programs for service members / editors,
George B. Meyers and Alice M. Glaskin.
p. ; cm.
Includes bibliographical references and index.
ISBN 978-1-61209-581-3 (hardcover : alk. paper)
1. Veterans--Medical care--United States. 2. Veterans--Service
for--United States. 3. Disabled veterans--Medical care--United States. 4.
Disabled veterans--Services for--United States. I. Meyers, George B. II.
Glaskin, Alice M.
[DNLM: 1. Veterans Health--United States. 2. Veterans Disability
Claims--United States. WA 360]
UB369.V474 2011
362.860973--dc22
2011004285

Published by Nova Science Publishers, Inc. † New York

AGING ISSUES, HEALTH AND FINANCIAL ALTERNATIVES

VETERANS BENEFITS: A SELECTION OF PROGRAMS FOR SERVICE MEMBERS

Aging Issues, Health and Financial Alternatives

Additional books in this series can be found on Nova's website under the Series tab.

Additional E-books in this series can be found on Nova's website under the E-books tab.

Health Care Issues, Costs and Access

Additional books in this series can be found on Nova's website under the Series tab.

Additional E-books in this series can be found on Nova's website under the E-books tab.

CONTENTS

PREFACE

The Department of Veterans Affairs (VA) administers directly, or in conjunction with other federal agencies, programs that provide benefits and other services to veterans and their spouses, dependents and beneficiaries. This new book outlines a selection of benefits for service members, including Dependency and Indemnity Compensation (DIC) for survivors of certain service members and veterans; healthcare for dependents and survivors of veterans; benefits for service-connected disabilities; project HERO implementation; health care and benefits for veterans exposed to agent orange and veterans life insurance programs.

Chapter 1- The Department of Veterans Affairs (VA) administers directly, or in conjunction with other federal agencies, programs that provide benefits and other services to veterans and their spouses, dependents, and beneficiaries.

One of the benefits administered by the VA is Dependency and Indemnity Compensation (DIC) for survivors of certain servicemembers and veterans. DIC is a monthly tax-free cash payment to survivors and dependents of servicemembers killed while on active military duty, and for survivors and dependents of certain veterans. Survivors of veterans who die from service-related conditions are eligible for DIC. Survivors of veterans who die from non-service-connected conditions may be eligible for DIC if the veteran was eligible for, or was receiving, disability compensation as totally disabled (a 100% rating) for a period of time (specified in statute) before the veteran's death.

Chapter 2- The Civilian Health and Medical Program of the Department of Veterans Affairs (CHAMPVA) is primarily a fee-for-service program that provides reimbursement for most medical care for certain eligible dependents and survivors of veterans rated permanently and totally disabled from a service-connected condition. This chapter provides an overview of CHAMPVA and includes a series of questions and answers about the program.

Chapter 3- Congress provides various benefits to American veterans and their dependents through the United States Department of Veterans Affairs (VA). One of these benefits is *disability compensation*, which is a monthly cash benefit program for veterans currently impaired from past service-connected activities.

A claim for disability compensation is initially analyzed by the VA at the local level to determine (1) whether the claimant is considered a "veteran" (eligible for benefits); (2) whether the veteran qualifies for disability compensation (entitled to benefits); (3) the extent of the impairment and the "rate" of the disability; and (4) the effective date for the compensation.

Chapter 4- Although U.S. Armed Forces are deployed around the globe, a number of servicemembers are currently serving in the Operation Enduring Freedom (OEF) and Operation Iraq Freedom (OIF) combat zones. As a result of the risks facing these servicemembers, some of them are incurring injuries or illnesses during their active service (or having existing medical conditions worsen as a result of their service). Congress has shown an interest in the treatment of injured servicemembers while undergoing medical treatment and their transition from military to civilian life as veterans. An injured servicemember (or veteran) may require specific types of assistance or benefits to enable him or her to have a better quality of life.

Chapter 5- In general, the Department of Veterans Affairs (VA), through the Veterans Health Administration (VHA), provides a majority of medical services to veterans within its health care system. However, in some instances, such as when a clinical service cannot be provided by a VA medical center, when a veteran is unable to access VA health care facilities due to geographic inaccessibility, or in emergencies when delays could lead to life threatening situations, VHA is authorized by law to send the veteran outside of VA's health care system to seek care. In 2006, the conference report to accompany the Military Quality of Life and Veterans Affairs Appropriations Act of 2006 (P.L. 109-114, H.Rept. 109-305) directed the VA to implement a cost-effective purchased care management program and to develop at least three pilot programs to encourage collaboration with industry and academia. In response to this requirement, VHA established a demonstration program to enhance the existing fee basis care program that was named Project HERO (Healthcare Effectiveness through Resource Optimization).

Chapter 6- Since the 1970s, Vietnam-era veterans have attributed certain medical illnesses, disabilities, and birth defects to exposure to Agent Orange and other herbicides sprayed by the U.S. Air Force to destroy enemy crops and remove forest cover. During the last 30 years, Agent Orange legislation has established and updated the health and disability benefits of Vietnam veterans exposed to herbicides.

Chapter 7- The Department of Veterans Affairs (VA) administers and supervises several life insurance programs for active servicemembers and veterans. The VA supervises the Servicemembers' Group Life Insurance (SGLI) and Veterans' Group Life Insurance (VGLI) programs, which are administered by the Office of Servicemembers' Group Life Insurance (OSGLI), a division of Prudential Financial. The Service-Disabled Veterans' Insurance (S-DVI) program, on the other hand, is administered entirely by the VA. Access to VA-administered life insurance programs gives servicemembers and veterans, who may not be eligible for private life insurance policies, the opportunity to carry group life insurance. This provides for their families in the event of the servicemember's or veteran's death.

Chapter 8- There are federal employment and training programs and policies specifically targeted to help veterans seeking employment in the civilian economy. Transition assistance programs are operated by the Department of Defense (DOD), the Department of Veterans Affairs (VA), and the Department of Labor (DOL) to assist servicemembers as they prepare to leave the military. DOL operates grant programs to states to provide outreach and assistance to veterans in finding civilian employment. In addition, the federal government has policies (including veterans preference) that assist veterans in obtaining jobs with the federal government and federal contractors. This chapter provides a brief overview of these federal programs and policies.

Chapter 9- The number of servicemembers, National Guard, and Reservists who separate from active duty with service-connected disabilities is expected to rise as a result of the engagement of the U.S. Armed Forces in Operation Iraqi Freedom and Operation Enduring Freedom. There is concern in Congress that these individuals receive the care and services that will enable them to transition successfully back to civilian life. These veterans must be able to rejoin their families and communities, become employed, and continue to enjoy the highest quality of life possible, given their disabilities.

Chapter 10- The U.S. Department of Veterans Affairs (VA), previously named the Veterans Administration, has been providing veterans educational assistance benefits since 1944. The benefits have been intended, at various times, to compensate for compulsory service, encourage voluntary service, avoid unemployment, provide equitable benefits to all who served, and promote military retention. The categories of individuals eligible to receive benefits has expanded from just veterans to include service members, Reservists, National Guard members, and their dependents. Although the programs are administered by the VA, the Department of Defense pays certain benefits and provides additional benefits to certain persons with critical skills or lengthy service.

Chapter 11- The Department of Veterans Affairs (VA) administers several pension benefit programs for veterans as well as their surviving spouses and dependent children. The most current pension programs available (for those meeting the eligibility criteria on or after January 1, 1979) are the Improved Disability Pension for certain low-income veterans and the Improved Death Pension for certain low-income surviving spouses or children of veterans. There is also a special pension for Medal of Honor recipients. This chapter describes these programs, including the eligibility criteria and current benefit levels.

Chapter 12- Burial benefits are monetary and nonmonetary benefits that eligible veterans receive for their military service. Nonmonetary burial benefits have been provided to servicemembers and veterans since the Civil War. Monetary burial benefits have been provided to servicemembers and veterans since World War I.

In: Veterans Benefits
Editors: George B. Meyers and Alice M. Glaskin
ISBN: 978-1-61209-581-3

Chapter 1

VETERANS' BENEFITS: DEPENDENCY AND INDEMNITY COMPENSATION (DIC) FOR SURVIVORS

Christine Scott

SUMMARY

The Department of Veterans Affairs (VA) administers directly, or in conjunction with other federal agencies, programs that provide benefits and other services to veterans and their spouses, dependents, and beneficiaries.

One of the benefits administered by the VA is Dependency and Indemnity Compensation (DIC) for survivors of certain servicemembers and veterans. DIC is a monthly tax-free cash payment to survivors and dependents of servicemembers killed while on active military duty, and for survivors and dependents of certain veterans. Survivors of veterans who die from service-related conditions are eligible for DIC. Survivors of veterans who die from non-service-connected conditions may be eligible for DIC if the veteran was eligible for, or was receiving, disability compensation as totally disabled (a 100% rating) for a period of time (specified in statute) before the veteran's death.

Several policy issues are associated with DIC, including the DIC offset of Survivor Benefit Plan (military retirement survivor) payments, often referred to as the "widow's tax"; adequacy of the payments for survivors compared with other retirement systems payments to surviving spouses; the remarriage age of 57; length of time for a totally disabled rating for non-service-connected deaths to qualify for DIC; and maximum DIC payment for parents based on income levels that have not been adjusted for inflation.

This chapter outlines the eligibility requirements and benefit levels for DIC and related policy issues. Legislation has been introduced in the 111th Congress related to the issues discussed in this chapter. Although none of the bills introduced have seen legislative action, an amendment (S.Amdt. 1515) to S. 1390 was adopted on the Senate floor.

The Department of Veterans Affairs (VA) offers directly, or in conjunction with other federal agencies, several benefits for surviving spouses, children, and dependent parents of deceased veterans to provide them with financial, educational, and emotional support. Among these various programs, Dependency and Indemnity Compensation (DIC) is a monthly tax-free cash payment for eligible surviving spouses, children, and dependent parents.

DIC has been paid in some form (monthly cash payments or insurance benefits) to survivors since the Revolutionary War. There were modifications after each war until the 1950s, when the federal government mandated a more streamlined process that created the system used currently for survivors of veterans and military servicemen.

Several policy issues are associated with DIC, including the DIC offset of Survivor Benefit Plan (military retirement survivor) payments, often referred to as the "widow's tax"; adequacy of the payments for surviving spouses compared with the payments made by retirement systems to surviving spouses; remarriage age of 57; length of time for a totally disabled rating for nonservice-connected deaths to qualify for DIC; and maximum DIC payment for parents based on income levels that have not been adjusted for inflation.

This chapter outlines the eligibility requirements and benefit levels for DIC, the policy issues associated with DIC, and legislation in the 111th Congress related to DIC.

ELIGIBILITY REQUIREMENTS

The eligibility for DIC by survivors is based on (1) the eligibility of the veteran, which is determined by the circumstances of the veteran's death and his or her disability compensation rating; and (2) the survivor meeting certain criteria related to either relationship to the veteran, age, or income.

Veteran Eligibility

The recipients of DIC must be the survivors of qualifying veterans. By statute, a "veteran" is defined as a "person who served in the active military, naval, or air service, and who was discharged or released therefrom under conditions other than dishonorable." DIC is paid to eligible survivors for three categories of veterans whose deaths fit one of the following circumstances:

1. veterans who died on active duty,[1] active duty for training, or inactive duty for training;
2. veterans who died due to service-connected disabilities;[2] or
3. veterans who died from non-service-related causes not as a result of willful misconduct and were receiving, or eligible to receive, disability compensation from the VA for service-connected disabilities rated at 100% subject to the following stipulations:[3]
    - the disabilities were rated as 100% disabled for 10 years or more prior to death;
    - the disabilities were rated as 100% since discharge or release from active duty for at least five years prior to death; or
    - the veterans were prisoners of war who had service-connected disabilities rated at 100% for at least one year prior to death after September 30, 1999.[4]

The Veterans' Benefits Act of 2010 (P.L. 111-275) expanded the criteria for survivors of veterans who were prisoners of war and died from non-service-related causes by eliminating the requirement that the veteran had to have service-connected disabilities rated at 100% disabled for one year prior to death.

The VA determines the eligibility of veterans and their entitlement to disability compensation through evidence found in military department service records and circumstances of death.[5]

WHAT IS A "VETERAN" FOR THE PURPOSES OF VA BENEFITS?

Federal statutes define "veteran" as a "person who served in the active military, naval, or air service, and who was discharged or released there from under conditions other than dishonorable." [38 U.S.C. § 101(2); 38 C.F.R. § 3.1(d)]. The VA largely bases its determination of veteran status upon military department service records. In addition to the member's service records, other factors affect his or her classification as a "veteran" and may affect future benefits. These factors include the following:

- *Discharge criteria:* (38 U.S.C. § 101(2); 38 C.F.R. § 3.1(d)).
- *Active military, naval or air service:* (38 U.S.C. § 101(2); 38 C.F.R. § 3.1(d)).
- *Whether the service was during "time of war:"* (38 U.S.C. § 101(6)-(1 1); 38 C.F.R. § 3.2).
- *Minimum active-duty service requirement:* (38 U.S.C. § 5303A 38, C.F.R. § 3.1 2A).

After it has been proved that the discharged servicemember meets these criteria, he or she is considered to be a "veteran," and may be eligible for certain benefits relating to health care, education, and other services provided by the VA.

(Information provided by Douglas Reid Weimer, legislative attorney, American Law Division, CRS.)

Recipient Eligibility

The dependents of veterans are not generally entitled to all benefits administered by the VA, but some benefits are available based on the relationship the dependent may have had with the veteran. If the eligibility criteria for DIC related to the veteran's death are met, the survivors also have certain criteria to meet to be eligible for DIC. There are three different groups of recipients: spouses, children, and dependent parents of deceased veterans. Each group has specific eligibility requirements.

Surviving Spouses

A surviving spouse is eligible if he or she

- was married to the veteran for at least one year before the veteran's death,[6] or

- has a child with the veteran, or
- if the veteran left the military due to a service-connected disability, the marriage was within 15 years of the discharge;
- cohabited with the veteran for the duration of the marriage unless the couple underwent a period of separation that was not the fault of the surviving spouse; and
- has not remarried before reaching the age of 57.[7]

Surviving Children

Surviving children[8] are eligible for DIC if they are independent of the surviving spouse, unmarried, and below the age of 18. If they are aged 18 to 23, they must be pursuing an approved course of education to be eligible for DIC.[9] Children who are permanently incapable of supporting themselves at the age of 18 or older remain entitled to DIC.[10]

Surviving Parents

Surviving parents are required to provide evidence of financial dependence on the deceased veteran before becoming eligible for DIC. This evidence is gained through a calculation of countable income[11] by the VA that cannot exceed the amounts outlined in the Income for VA Purposes (IVAP) tables.[12]

MONTHLY BENEFIT AMOUNTS

Surviving Spouses

Surviving spouses receive monthly benefits at a current base rate of $1,154 if the veteran died on or after January 1, 1993.[13] Otherwise, payment is based on the veteran's pay grade at the time of death with the current lowest rate being $1,154.[14] A higher amount may be provided to the surviving spouse for several reasons:

- if the veteran, eight years before death was receiving or entitled to receive disability compensation for a service-connected disability rated at totally disabled (100%);
- if the surviving spouse has dependent children; or
- if the surviving spouse has a disability that requires aid and assistance or is permanently housebound.

If all of these factors are considered, a surviving spouse could currently receive a total of up to $1,686, along with $286 for each dependent child under the age of 18.[15] There is also an additional benefit provided for spouses with dependent children under 18 for a two-year period or until the children reach 18 years of age to ease the transition of the surviving spouse and children to their new income levels.[16]

Surviving Children

Surviving children under the age of 18, or under the age of 23 if they are students, who are independent of the surviving spouse, are entitled to DIC in the following current monthly amounts: one child receives $488, two children receive $701, three children receive $915 and more than three children receive $915 with an additional $174 for each additional child past three. If a child is permanently incapable of self-support before the age of 18, the child remains eligible for DIC past the age of 18.

Surviving Parents

Under current law, the maximum allowable DIC for surviving dependent parents is reduced for countable income above $800, or $1,000 if both parents are a married couple. Monthly benefits received by parents fluctuate by income. [17] In the case of a sole surviving parent, the monthly DIC benefit ranges between $5 and $569. For parents who are still married to each other or have remarried other individuals, the range is between $5 and $387. For parents who are not living with each other or different spouses, the range is between $5 and $412.

Application Process

To claim DIC benefits, a survivor is to complete and submit to the local VA office VA Form 21- 534a and Department of Defense (DD) Form 1300, Report of Casualty.[18] The effective date of DIC entitlement is the first day of the month that the death occurred for claims filed within one year of the death. After one year, the DIC entitlement starts on the date the claim is received by the VA.[19]

Use of DIC in FY2008

In FY2008, 320,975 spouses, children, and parents of veterans received more than $4.6 billion in DIC.[20] On average, each survivor received $13,938 in annual compensation. Children recipients received an average of $6,662 in annual compensation.[21] **Table 1** shows DIC recipients by state and category for FY2008.

Policy Issues Related to DIC

Several policy issues are associated with DIC, including the DIC offset of Survivor Benefit Plan (military retirement survivor) payments, often referred to as the "widow's tax"; adequacy of the payments for survivors compared to other retirement systems' payments to surviving spouses; remarriage age of 57;

Table 1. DIC Recipients by State and Category for FY2008

State	Spouses	Children	Parents	Total
Alabama	8,342	706	200	9,248
Alaska	587	99	7	693
Arizona	7,226	545	61	7,832
Arkansas	5,303	434	114	5,851
California	27,796	2,117	334	30,247
Colorado	5,510	489	51	6,050
Connecticut	1,866	111	16	1,993
Delaware	887	88	10	985
District of Columbia	517	38	17	572
Florida	26,952	1,738	298	28,988
Georgia	13,296	1,346	258	14,900
Hawaii	1,641	160	22	1,823
Idaho	1,509	135	13	1,657
Illinois	5,844	553	110	6,507
Indiana	4,438	425	63	4,926
Iowa	2,244	221	22	2,487
Kansas	2,863	295	30	3,188
Kentucky	5,379	569	109	6,057
Louisiana	5,082	471	158	5,711
Maine	1,898	136	37	2,071
Maryland	5,407	509	63	5,979
Massachusetts	5,899	378	50	6,327
Michigan	6,711	678	107	7,496
Minnesota	3,918	282	50	4,250
Mississippi	4,194	400	147	4,741
Missouri	6,030	495	80	6,605
Montana	1,080	127	9	1,216
Nebraska	1,971	149	27	2,147
Nevada	2,596	197	6	2,799
New Hampshire	1,345	72	7	1,424
New Jersey	5,278	370	45	5,693
New Mexico	2,919	236	66	3,221
New York	10,493	893	218	11,604
North Carolina	13,643	1,452	320	15,415
North Dakota	577	74	10	661
Ohio	8,835	806	151	9,792
Oklahoma	7,355	585	87	8,027
Oregon	4,146	322	21	4,489
Pennsylvania	10,468	851	144	11,463
Puerto Rico	2,961	322	273	3,556
Rhode Island	1,115	93	11	1,219
South Carolina	7,111	632	157	7,900
South Dakota	950	89	11	1,050
Tennessee	8,171	772	181	9,124
Texas	29,619	2,708	442	32,769
Utah	1,501	214	16	1,731
Vermont	616	53	9	678
Virginia	12,262	1,248	132	13,642
Washington	8,759	694	55	9,508
West Virginia	2,717	251	43	3,011
Wisconsin	3,964	337	49	4,350
Wyoming	543	42	5	590
Territories & Other	8,641	1,009	203	9,853
U.S. Total	320,975	28,016	5,125	354,116

Source: Table prepared by the Congressional Research Service (CRS) using data from the Department of Veterans Affairs (VA).

length of time for a totally disabled rating for non-service-connected deaths to qualify for DIC; and maximum DIC payment for parents based on income levels that have not been adjusted for inflation.

Related legislation has been introduced in the 111th Congress. Although none of the bills introduced have seen legislative action, an amendment (S.Amdt. 1515) to S. 1390 was adopted on the Senate floor, which would eliminate the DIC/SBP offset (described below).

DIC and SBP Offset

The Survivor Benefit Plan (SBP) is a form of insurance provided by the Department of Defense to military retirees that does not require service-connected death or disability for survivors to receive payments.[22] A military retiree elects to have lower monthly retirement pay—the insurance premium for SBP is taken from retirement pay—to ensure that his or her survivors can receive a monthly payment after his or her death. However, this income is taxable, while DIC is tax-free. If the survivor of a military retiree is also eligible for and receives DIC, the SBP payment is reduced dollar for dollar by the DIC amount (but not below zero).

DIC Percentage of Income Compared with Other Pension Programs

There is a disparity between the percentage of income a DIC recipient is paid and the percentages given to recipients of retirement and pension plans. Currently, an eligible surviving spouse would receive a basic DIC benefit of $1,154 monthly. This is 40.8% of the basic compensation rate for a veteran with a spouse receiving disability compensation at the 100% disabled rating. This has called into question the adequacy of DIC payments.

Private pension plans are required to pay 50% of their benefit to surviving spouses, but retirees in some plans may elect to give their surviving spouses a larger percentage. As a result of the variance in pension plans, benefits, and survivor options, it is difficult to discern what the average pension benefit for a surviving spouse in the private sector might be. SBP recipients receive 55% of the military retiree's retirement pay.[23] Federal employee pension plans provide 55% of retirement pay, or 50% of retirement pay along with an initial lump-sum payment, depending on the plan.[24]

Low-income elderly or disabled veterans may be eligible for the Improved Disability Pension. In the event of their death, the surviving spouse may be eligible for the Improved Death Pension Benefit. The surviving spouse would receive, under the Improved Death Pension, about 51.2% of the veteran's Improved Disability Pension benefit.[25]

As a percentage of 100% disability compensation, DIC is below the 50% or more level for survivors associated with other retirement or pension benefits. However, unlike pension benefits, DIC is not structured as a percentage of the disability compensation received by the veteran. Under the current DIC structure, the surviving spouse of a veteran who died with a disability rating of less than 70% would receive more in DIC than the veteran received in disability compensation while alive (based on the current disability compensation rates for a veteran with a spouse). If DIC were 50% of the disability compensation received by the veteran, a survivor would receive a basic monthly benefit (based on the veteran's disability rating) ranging from $62 to $1,412.[26] This range exists because a veteran could die from a service-connected condition that is rated at less than 100%. As a result, the surviving spouse could receive more from DIC ($1,154) than the veteran received from disability compensation.

DIC Remarriage Age

Until 2003, a surviving spouse could not remarry and continue to receive DIC benefits. That changed with the enactment of the Veterans Benefits Act of 2003 (P.L. 108-183), which allowed a surviving spouse at aged 57 or older to remarry and keep DIC benefits. For the military Survivor Benefit Plan and for federal employees, the remarriage age is 55 for retaining benefits, and for Social Security beneficiaries, the remarriage age is 60. The difference in ages for remarriage means that a remarried surviving spouse may not be able to keep all of his or her benefits if he or she remarries.

Disability Requirement for Non-Service-Connected Deaths

As stated earlier (see "Eligibility Requirements" section), if a veteran's death was not service- connected, the veteran must have been receiving, or been eligible to receive, disability compensation as 100% disabled for 10 years or more prior to death to enable a survivor to be eligible for DIC. Some totally disabled veterans have expressed concern that their surviving spouses would not receive a benefit if they die from non-service-connected causes if they have not been totally disabled for at least 10 years. The 10-year disability requirement for non-serviceconnected deaths can be viewed as a measure of the survivor's dependence on the veteran's disability compensation. This view assumes that the longer the veteran was disabled, the more dependent the survivors were on the veteran's disability compensation as a replacement of the veteran's earnings.

Maximum Benefit for Dependent Parents

For survivors, income is not a factor in DIC eligibility unless the survivor is a dependent parent. The maximum DIC amount payable to parents is only for parents below a stationary income level: $800 for a single parent and $1,000 for a married couple. These amounts were enacted into law in 1968 and unlike other income levels related to benefits, they have not been adjusted for inflation. The $800 limitation in 1968 is equivalent to $4,958 in 2009. This means that dependent parents over time may see reductions in DIC as their incomes increase due to cost of living adjustments in their other income, because the $800 and $1,000 income limitations for DIC are not adjusted for inflation.

LEGISLATIVE HISTORY

Dependency and indemnity compensation (DIC) has been paid in some form to survivors since the Revolutionary War. At that time, women and children survivors of officers received a seven- year pension amounting to half of the officer's entitled pay (according to a 1780 act of the Continental Congress).[27]

During the Civil War, survivor compensation was expanded to cover all servicemembers at a rate that would be payable to totally disabled veterans.[28] The Civil War also lead to other changes to survivor compensation, especially for survivors of servicemembers with service-connected disabilities. They were covered under the Act of July 14, 1862, which was referred to as General Law and amended various times in the 19th century.

In 1917, Congress passed the War Risk Insurance Act to eliminate the need for non-service pensions and highlighted that service-connected payments for death and disability were compensation payments.[29] The act changed the system to meet the current needs of World War I veterans and their survivors and eliminated the pay discrepancy between officers and soldiers.[30]

The Servicemen's Indemnity Act of 1951 replaced this life insurance system with a new system where the servicemembers did not contribute to the insurance program, but the government provided monthly payments to eligible survivors of $120 with a 2.25% increase per year until a $10,000 insurance maximum was reached.[31] Potentially eligible survivors included spouses, children, parents, and siblings.

Because legislation had been written in response to need, dependency and indemnity compensation was unorganized and administered by four different administrations by the mid- 1950s, and congressional and executive committees were formed to make the issuance of compensation more streamlined and manageable. [32] Death compensation was set up similar to the way it is now by the time the final report of the President's Commission on Veterans' Pensions, *Veterans' Benefits in the United States: Report to the President by the President's Commission of Veterans Pensions* (hereafter referred to as the Bradley Report) was written in 1956.[33] Death compensation was provided to survivors (except for dependent parents) regardless of income. The rate of compensation depended on whether the veteran served in peacetime or wartime.

In 1969, after review of the Bradley Report, recommendations from a commission headed by Robert M. McCurdy in 1967,[34] and extensive testimony from several other federal administrations and veterans service organizations, Congress devised a different, more equitable system for survivor compensation that gave fixed rates to each pay grade. The base rate was adjusted for a cost-of-living increase to reflect changes in the cost-of-living since the last base rate had been determined in 1956, 13 years earlier.[35] In 1969, years of service were no longer a factor in determining DIC.[36] There were no subsequent changes of significance to DIC legislation until 1993, when the rate tables for surviving spouses were eliminated and one flat monthly rate was reinstated.[37] In 2003, surviving spouses who remarried after reaching the age of 57 were able to retain DIC.[38]

ACKNOWLEDGMENTS

This chapter was written by Jayla L. Randleman, a former intern with the Congressional Research Service. All questions should be directed to the current author.

End Notes

[1] Active duty is considered to include (1) full-time service in the Army, Navy, Marine Corps, Air Force, or Coast Guard, other than active duty for training (38 U.S.C. § 101(21)(A); 38 C.F.R. § 3.6(b)(1)); (2) full-time service as a commissioned officer in the Public Health Service (38 U.S.C. § 101(21)(B); 38 C.F.R. § 3.6(b)(2)); (3) full-time service as a commissioned officer at the Coast and Geodetic Survey, Environmental Services Administration, or National Oceanic and Atmospheric Administration (38 U.S.C. § 101(21)(C); 38 C.F.R. § 3.6(b)(3)); (4) service as a cadet at a military academy (38 U.S.C. § 101(21)(D); 38 C.F.R. § 3.6(b)(4)); (5) attendance by active-duty members at certain prep schools associated with military academies (38 C.F.R. § 3.6(b)(5)); and (6) authorized travel to or from such duty or service (38 U.S.C. § 101(21)(E); 38 C.F.R. § 3.6(b)(6)).

[2] A service-connected disability is defined in 38 U.S.C. §101(16).

[3] Eligibility for non-service-connected deaths of certain veterans rated totally disabled was added by P.L. 100-687.

[4] 38 U.S.C. § 1318.

[5] For more information regarding VA disability requirements, see CRS Report RL33 113, *Veterans Affairs: Basic Eligibility for Disability Benefit Programs*, by Douglas Reid Weimer.

[6] This requirement does not exist for surviving spouses of a servicemember killed on active military duty.

[7] Congress passed the Veterans' Benefits Act of 2003, which allowed surviving spouse to remarry after the age of 57. P.L. 108-183; 38 U.S.C §§103, 1304.

[8] Definitions of who is considered a child for the purpose of VA benefits are outlined in 38 U.S.C § 101 (4).

[9] Students receiving DIC are not able to concurrently receive education benefits under the G.I. Bill or from the VA Survivors' and Dependents Educational Assistance Program under 38 USC § 3562.

[10] 38 U.S.C §§ 1313, 1314.

[11] Exclusions for countable income are outlined in 38 CFR § 3.272, available at http://law.justia.com/us/cfr/title38/38- 1.0.1.1.4.1.62.101.html.

[12] The applicable rate table can be found at VA's website, at http://www.vba.va.gov/bln /21/Rates/comp04.htm#BMC1.

[13] All benefits listed are adjusted for cost of living expenses coinciding with the percentage decided for Social Security benefits in accordance with 38 U.S.C § 1303.

[14] See rate tables at http://www.vba.va.gov/bln/21/Rates/comp03.htm#BM03.

[15] See http://www1.va.gov/opa/Is1/11.asp.

[16] 38 U.S.C § 1311(f).

[17] To see income level rate charts, visit http://www.vba.va.gov/BLN/21/Rates/comp04.htm#BMC3.

[18] To download VA Form 21-534a, go to this link, http://www.vba.va.gov/survivors. For parental DIC, download VA Form 21-535 at http://www.vba.va.gov/pubs/forms/21-535.pdf. The Department of Defense Form 1300 is located at http://www.dtic.mil/whs/directives

[19] 38 U.S.C § 5110.

[20] Department of Veterans Affairs, *Annual Benefits Report FY2008*, available at http://www.vba.va.g ov/REPORTS/abr/ 2008_abr.pdf.

[21] Ibid.

[22] For more information on the Survivor Benefit Plan, see CRS Report RL32769, *Military Death Benefits: Status and Proposals*, by David F. Burrelli and Jennifer R. Corwell.

[23] For additional information regarding veterans pension programs, see CRS Report RS22804, *Veterans' Benefits: Pension Benefit Programs*, by Christine Scott and Carol D. Davis.

[24] For more information on survivor benefits for federal employees, see CRS Report RS2 1029, *Survivor Benefits for Families of Civilian Federal Employees and Retirees*, by Katelin P. Isaacs.

[25] If both pension payments were received at their maximum rates (which would be dependent on income levels).

[26] Fifty percent of the disability compensation for a veteran with a spouse.

[27] Omar N. Bradley, Clarence G. Adamy, and William J. Donovan, et al., *Veterans' Benefits in the United States: A Report to President by the President's Commission on Veterans' Pensions*, The Bradley Commission, Washington DC, April 1956. (Hereafter referred to as the Bradley Report.)

[28] Ibid.

[29] P.L. 65-105.

[30] Ibid.
[31] P.L. 82-23.
[32] Sen. Bob Graham, "Honor the DIC commitment," remarks in the Senate, *Congressional Record*, vol. 137 (November 12, 1991), pp. S16332-S16338.
[33] Bradley Report (Washington DC: April 1956), pp. 33-52.
[34] Sen. Bob Graham, "Honor the DIC commitment," remarks in the Senate, *Congressional Record*, vol. 137 (November 12, 1991), pp. 31116-31123.
[35] Ibid.
[36] Ibid.
[37] P.L. 102-568.
[38] P.L. 108-183.

In: Veterans Benefits
Editors: George B. Meyers and Alice M. Glaskin
ISBN: 978-1-61209-581-3

Chapter 2

HEALTH CARE FOR DEPENDENTS AND SURVIVORS OF VETERANS

Sidath Viranga Panangala

SUMMARY

The Civilian Health and Medical Program of the Department of Veterans Affairs (CHAMPVA) is primarily a fee-for-service program that provides reimbursement for most medical care for certain eligible dependents and survivors of veterans rated permanently and totally disabled from a service-connected condition. This chapter provides an overview of CHAMPVA and includes a series of questions and answers about the program.

OVERVIEW

The Veterans Health Administration (VHA) of the Department of Veterans Affairs (VA) provides health care services to veterans who meet certain eligibility requirements. The VHA is primarily a direct service provider of primary care, specialized care, and related medical and social support services to veterans though an integrated health care system. In 1973, Congress established the Civilian Health and Medical Program of the Department of Veterans Affairs (CHAMPVA) as a means of providing health care services to dependents and survivors of certain veterans.[1] As stated in the House report accompanying P.L. 93-82:

> The nation has long recognized that the widow and children of a veteran who dies of service- connected disease or injury or of a veteran who has a service-connected total disability are in a special category and deserving of substantial compensation and assistance in return for the sacrifice the family has made. This recognition has been shown in title 38 programs which provide for death compensation benefits, home loans, and educational assistance benefits for wives, widows, and war orphans. Failure to provide for the medical care of such individuals is an oversight which should be corrected.[2]

CHAMPVA primarily is a fee-for-service program that provides reimbursement for most medical care for certain eligible dependents and survivors of veterans rated permanently and totally disabled from a service-connected condition.[3] CHAMPVA is a cost-sharing program that reimburses providers and facilities a determined allowable amount, minus patient co-pay and deductible. CHAMPVA was designed to provide medical care in a manner similar to the care provided to certain eligible beneficiaries under the Department of Defense (DOD) TRICARE program (see the description below). The number of beneficiaries enrolled in CHAMPVA has grown over the years. From FY2001 through FY2009, enrollment grew by 248%—from 96,500 to 336,300 beneficiaries (see **Figure 1**). The 2001 expansion of CHAMP VA eligibility to certain individuals aged 65 years and older has contributed to the increase in enrollment. Moreover, there has been an increase in enrollment of dependents and spouses of certain Vietnam-era veterans with service-connected disabilities. This increase in Vietnam-era CHAMPVA sponsorship has occurred as aging Vietnam-era veterans with service-connected disabilities experience a worsening of symptoms and a change in disability status. Once a veteran becomes VA-rated permanently and totally disabled for a service-connected disability, the veteran's spouse and dependents are then eligible to enroll in CHAMP VA.

Moreover, the number of unique CHAMP VA users has grown by 277% from FY200 1 to FY2009 (see **Figure 2**). Unique users are enrollees who utilize a health benefit at least once in a fiscal year.

Funding for CHAMPVA is provided through the VHA's Medical Services account.[4] As shown in **Table 1**, spending for CHAMPVA grew steadily in the past eight years. Between FY2002 and FY2009, CHAMPVA expenditures increased by 336%, while the number of unique users increased by only 187% during the same period. These data imply an increased average cost per patient from approximately $2,495 per patient in FY2002 to $3,791 per patient in FY2009. A demographic shift in CHAMP VA enrollees from less expensive younger beneficiaries to more expensive aging beneficiaries, in addition to the general inflation of medical costs, has contributed to the increase in CHAMP VA expenditures.

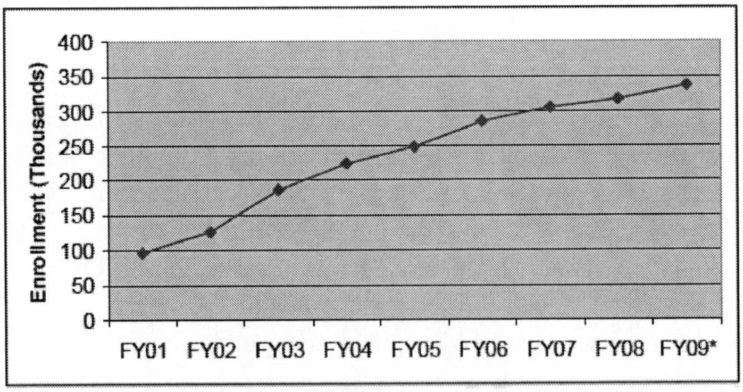

Source: Chart prepared by Congressional Research Service (CRS), based on data from the Department of Veterans Affairs.

* These are the estimated enrolled beneficiaries for FY2009.

Figure 1. CHAMPVA-Enrolled Beneficiaries, FY200 1 -FY2009.

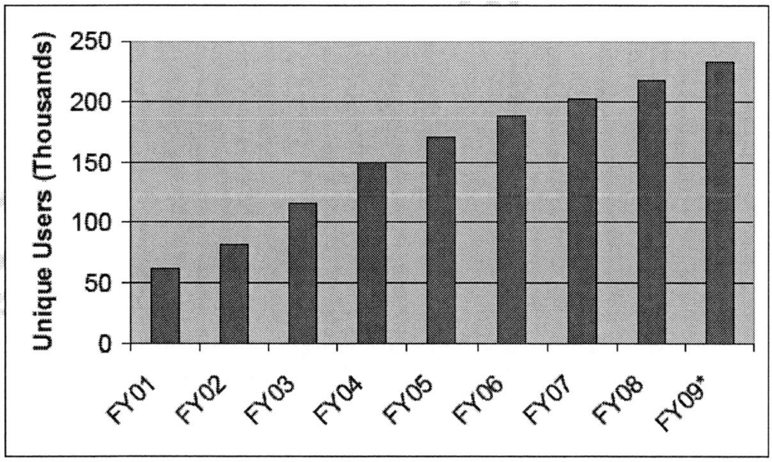

Source: Chart prepared by Congressional Research Service (CRS), based on data from the Department of Veterans Affairs.
* These are the estimated enrolled beneficiaries for FY2009.

Figure 2. CHAMPVA Unique Users, FY2002-FY2009.

Table 1. CHAMPVA Expenditures, FY2002-FY2009 ($ in Millions)

	FY2002 Actual	FY2003 Actual	FY2004 Actual	FY2005 Actual	FY2006 Actual	FY2007 Actual	FY2008 Actual	FY2009 Actual
Expenditures	$203.1	$318.2	$454.5	$565.5	$656.9	$712.2	$794.0	$885.2

Source: Table prepared by Congressional Research Service (CRS), based on data from the U.S. Department of Veterans Affairs, *Congressional Budget Submissions (FY2004-11), Medical Programs*.

The next section provides answers to frequently asked questions about the program.

QUESTIONS AND ANSWERS[5]

Who Is Eligible to Receive CHAMPVA Benefits?

Eligibility for CHAMPVA requires inclusion in one of the following categories:[6]

- the individual is the spouse or child of a veteran who has been rated permanently and totally disabled for a service-connected disability;
- the individual is the surviving spouse or child of a veteran who died from a VA-rated service-connected disability;
- the individual is the surviving spouse or child of a veteran who was at the time of death rated permanently and totally disabled from a service-connected disability; or

- the individual is the surviving spouse or child of a military member who died on active duty, not due to misconduct (in most cases, these family members are eligible under TRICARE, not CHAMPVA).

What Happens if a CHAMPVA-Eligible Spouse Divorces or Remarries?

CHAMPVA eligibility is terminated by divorce or annulment of marriage to the qualifying veteran. CHAMPVA has specific eligibility rules for widows. When a CHAMPVA-eligible widow remarries, eligibility is terminated if the marriage occurs before the age of 55. As of February 4, 2003, a CHAMP VA-eligible widow who remarries at age 55 or older remains eligible for CHAMPVA. If a CHAMP VA-eligible widow under the age of 55 remarries, and the remarriage is later terminated, the widow is again eligible for CHAMPVA.

When Does a Child Lose Eligibility?

In general, eligibility for CHAMP VA is lost when either a child (other than a helpless child)[7] turns 18, unless enrolled in an accredited school as a full-time student; a child, who has been a full-time student, turns 23 or loses full-time student status; a child marries; or a stepchild no longer lives in the household of the sponsor.

What Is the Difference between CHAMPVA and TRICARE?

Before distinguishing between the two programs, it is important to make the distinction between a veteran and a military retiree. Title 38 of the United States Code defines a "veteran" as a person who has been discharged under conditions other than dishonorable from active military, naval, or air service.[8] All military retirees, by definition, are veterans. However, to be considered a "military retiree," an individual generally must have spent at least 20 years on active duty in the armed services. CHAMPVA is a comprehensive program run by the VA for eligible family members of veterans rated permanently and totally disabled for a service-connected disability or the family members of veterans who died from a VA-rated service-connected disability. The sponsoring veteran does not receive services through CHAMP VA, as he or she is eligible to receive services through the VA. Dependents of military retirees are not eligible for CHAMPVA, and must apply for benefits through TRICARE. TRICARE is a health care program run by the DOD for families of active duty military service members, families of service members who died while on active duty, and retired military service men, women, and their families, regardless of their disability status. TRICARE has no disability criteria required for eligibility.[9]

What Is the Relationship of CHAMPVA and Medicare?

Under section three of the Veterans' Survivors Benefits Improvement Act of 2001, referred to as CHAMPVA for Life (P.L. 107-14), CHAMPVA benefits were expanded to those over the age of 65 in the following circumstances. CHAMPVA is the secondary payer for beneficiaries with Medicare coverage.

- If a beneficiary turns 65 before June 5, 2001, and only receives Medicare Part A, the beneficiary is eligible for CHAMPVA without having to purchase Medicare Part B coverage.
- If a beneficiary turns 65 before June 5, 2001, and receives both Medicare Part A and Part B, the beneficiary must retain both parts to be eligible for continued CHAMP VA as secondary coverage.
- If a beneficiary turns 65 on or after June 5, 2001, the beneficiary must be enrolled in Medicare Parts A and B to be eligible for CHAMP VA.
- Enrollment in Medicare Part D is not required to become or remain eligible for CHAMP VA.
- Individuals aged 65 or older not entitled to Medicare Part A retain CHAMP VA eligibility.

What Happens if the Beneficiary Has Other Health Insurance?

By law, CHAMPVA is generally the secondary payer for beneficiaries having any other form of health insurance. The primary health insurance company is billed first, and then beneficiaries submit an explanation of benefits (EOB) for additional reimbursement by CHAMP VA. The exception is for beneficiaries with Medicaid, beneficiaries receiving care under the State Victims of Crime Compensation Program, or beneficiaries with a CHAMP VA supplementary insurance policy. In those cases, CHAMPVA is the first payer. [10]

What Medical Benefits Are Available to Eligible Beneficiaries?

The CHAMPVA program covers most health care services and supplies that are determined to be medically necessary, including inpatient and outpatient care, prescription drugs, mental health services, and skilled nursing care. By law, CHAMPVA is required to provide health care benefits that are similar to the DOD's TRICARE program. Chiropractic services, routine eye examinations, hearing aids, and most dental benefits are excluded from both the federal CHAMPVA and TRICARE programs.[11] In late 2008, benefits were expanded to include any non- dental prostheses and removed the exclusion from coverage of enuretic (bed-wetting) devices. [12]

Certain types of care require advance approval, commonly know as preauthorization. Generally, a CHAMPVA beneficiary should ask a provider if the provider will accept a CHAMPVA beneficiary. This is known as "accepting assignment." What that means is the provider will bill the VA directly for covered services, items and supplies. They will be paid the "allowable charge." Doctors or providers who agree to accept assignment cannot try to collect more than the CHAMP VA deductible and cost share amounts from the beneficiary. If provider does not accept assignment, the CHAMP VA beneficiary is responsible for paying the annual deductible, the cost share amount (copay), and any provider-billed amount that exceeds our total allowable amount.

For care that is not covered by CHAMPVA, the beneficiary has to pay the full bill.[13] For example, with very few exceptions, dental care is not a covered benefit. Currently, preauthorization is required for

- durable medical equipment,
- hospice services,
- mental health/substance abuse services,
- organ and bone marrow transplants, and
- dental procedures that are directly related to covered medical conditions.

What Is the CHAMPVA Payment Structure?

CHAMPVA is a cost-sharing program that reimburses at rates comparable to the Medicare and TRICARE programs. CHAMPVA has an outpatient deductible of $50 per person and $100 per family per calendar year. After the deductible is reached, CHAMPVA pays 75% of the allowable amount, and the beneficiary pays 25% of the total amount. [14] The patient typically pays the cost share at the time the service is provided, unless the beneficiary has another health insurance plan. In cases where a beneficiary has another form of health insurance, CHAMPVA is the secondary payer (with the exception of the circumstances outlined in question five), and pays the lesser of either 75% of the allowable amount after the deductible or the rest of the billed charges. There is a $3,000 cap on cost sharing per CHAMPVA-eligible family. There is also an exception to the payment scheme outlined here for instances in which medical services are rendered through VA facilities participating in the CHAMPVA In-house Treatment Initiative (CITI).[15]

What Is the CHAMPVA In-House Treatment Initiative (CITI)?

The CITI is a voluntary program for CHAMP VA beneficiaries that provides medical care through local VA facilities on a space-available basis. Beneficiaries receiving care at the VA through the CITI program are not required to pay a deductible or participate in cost sharing. No extra enrollment is necessary to participate in the CITI program; the beneficiary simply has to determine if the local VA is a participating facility. The majority of VA facilities are CITI participants. It is important to emphasize that care is delivered based on the availability of space. Beneficiaries on Medicare or who have an HMO plan as their primary insurance are not eligible for the CITI program.

How Are CHAMPVA Claims Processed?

All CHAMPVA claims are processed through the VA Health Administration Center (HAC) in Denver, Colorado. Claims can be submitted by either the provider or the beneficiary, with each case requiring a different set of forms. All claims must be filed within one year after the date of service. For inpatient care, the claim must be filed within one year of the discharge date, and all payments will be made to the hospital regardless of which party submits the billing. Claims submitted after the one-year deadline will be denied. As of 2009, the ceiling on durable medical equipment (DME) was raised to $2,000 to facilitate the administrative claims process and to accurately reflect the current costs of medical equipment.[16]

End Notes

[1] Veterans Health Care Expansion Act of 1973 (P.L. 93-82).

[2] U.S. Congress, Committee on Veterans' Affairs, *Veterans Health Care Expansion Act of 1973*, report to accompany H.R. 9048, 93rd Congress, first session, H.Rept. 93-368 (Washington: GPO, 1973).

[3] The term "service-connected" means, with respect to disability, that such disability was incurred or aggravated in the line of duty in the active military, naval, or air service. VA determines whether veterans have service-connected disabilities, and for those with such disabilities, assigns ratings from 0 to 100% based on the severity of the disability. Percentages are assigned in increments of 10%.

[4] For detailed information on VHA appropriations, see CRS Report R40737, *Veterans Medical Care: FY2010 Appropriations*, by Sidath Viranga Panangala.

[5] This part was drawn from: Department of Veterans Affairs Health Administration Center, *CHAMPVA Handbook,* at http://www.va.gov/hac/forbeneficiaries/champva/handbook/chandbook.pdf and http://www4.va.gov/hac/forbeneficiaries/champva/champva.asp

[6] 38 U.S.C. § 1781; 38 C.F.R. § 17.270-17.278.

[7] A helpless child is established after a fact-based analysis completed by a VA Regional Office determines the child to be permanently incapable of self-support by the age of 18. See 38 C.F.R. § 3.356 and http://www.va.gov/hac/ forbeneficiaries/champva/handbook/chandbook.pdf.

[8] 38 U.S.C. § 101.

[9] For further information on TRICARE, see CRS Report RL33537, *Military Medical Care: Questions and Answers*, by Don J. Jansen. For specific provisions, see http://www.TRICARE.osd.mil; relevant regulations are at 32 C.F.R. § 199.

[10] 38 C.F.R. § 17.275.

[11] 38 C.F.R. § 17.272.

[12] Department of Veterans Affairs, "Civilian Health and Medical Program of the Department of Veterans Affairs (CHAMPVA): Expansion of Benefit Coverage for Prostheses and Enuretic Devices; Miscellaneous Provisions," 73 *Federal Register* 65552, November 4, 2008.

[13] Department of Veterans Affairs Health Administration Center. *Fact Sheet 01-16 for Outpatient Providers and Office Managers*. p. 1.

[14] An allowable amount is the maximum payment that is authorized by the VA for a covered medial service or supply.

[15] 38 C.F.R. § 17.274.

[16] Department of Veterans Affairs, "(CHAMPVA): Preauthorization of Durable Medical Equipment," 74 *Federal Register* 31373, July 1, 2009.

In: Veterans Benefits
Editors: George B. Meyers and Alice M. Glaskin
ISBN: 978-1-61209-581-3

Chapter 3

VETERANS AFFAIRS: BENEFITS FOR SERVICE-CONNECTED DISABILITIES

Douglas Reid Weimer

SUMMARY

Congress provides various benefits to American veterans and their dependents through the United States Department of Veterans Affairs (VA). One of these benefits is *disability compensation*, which is a monthly cash benefit program for veterans currently impaired from past service-connected activities.

A claim for disability compensation is initially analyzed by the VA at the local level to determine (1) whether the claimant is considered a "veteran" (eligible for benefits); (2) whether the veteran qualifies for disability compensation (entitled to benefits); (3) the extent of the impairment and the "rate" of the disability; and (4) the effective date for the compensation.

Three requirements to qualify for disability compensation are (1) medical diagnosis of the current impairment; (2) evidence of an in-service occurrence or an aggravation of the disease or injury; and (3) medical proof of a connection between the in-service incident or aggravation of an injury or illness and the current disability. The requisite standard of proof and certain medical presumptions are set by statute. The VA is required to provide assistance to the veteran in his/her case preparation by providing records and medical examinations. Special rules have been established for certain specific situations involving combat veterans, prisoners of war, and veterans exposed to Agent Orange.

If the veteran is found eligible for disability compensation, the VA then uses the Schedule for Rating Disabilities (SRD) to set the amount of earnings impairment on a percentage basis; the higher the percentage, the greater the compensation will be. Certain complications arise with the use of the rating system. A veteran's rating may be increased or decreased over time—depending on his/her medical condition. Rating decisions may be appealed administratively.

Legislation passed in the first session of the 111th Congress increased the 2010 monthly disability compensation payments by providing veterans a cost-of-living adjustment (COLA) for their VA benefits equal to the COLA for Social Security benefits (P.L. 111-37). However, in an unprecedented situation, no COLA for Social Security benefits was enacted. Therefore, there was no increase in the 2010 VA monthly disability compensation payments. The 111th Congress has considered additional legislation that may affect service-connected disabilities. Bills have been introduced to deal with the number of claims pending at the VA and issues related to the receipt of disability benefits. These include H.R. 3504 (the VA Case Backlog Alleviation and Economic Stimulus Act of 2009); H.R. 4121 (the Veterans Appeals Improvement and Modernization Act of 2009); S. 3286; S. 3348; S. 3368; S. 3370; S. 728; and H.R. 1037.

INTRODUCTION

Veterans' Disability Programs

Congress, through the United States Department of Veterans Affairs (VA), provides a wide variety of services and benefits to veterans and to certain members of their families.[1]

Two disability programs are administered by the VA. These programs pay monthly cash benefits to certain disabled veterans.[2] *Disability compensation*, the focus of this chapter, provides a monthly cash benefit if the veteran is at least 10% disabled as a consequence of his/her military service—which is considered to be a *service-connected disability*.[3] A veteran applying for service-connected disability compensation does not need to be totally disabled, have low income, or wartime military service. In contrast, a *disability pension* may be paid to a *wartime* veteran with limited income, who is no longer able to work, or is at least age 65.[4] A disability pension is not related to a service-connected injury or medical condition and takes into account the material needs of the veteran; it is a "needs-based" pension.[5]

The "Local Determination"

The VA analyzes each veteran's claim for disability compensation at the VA regional office closest to the veteran's residence, called the "local determination." This determination involves a four-step adjudication process of the veteran's claim.

First, the VA determines the claimant's basic eligibility to receive VA benefits. A determination is made as to whether the claimant was discharged or separated under other than dishonorable conditions, whether the claimant had "active service," and whether the claimant's condition is based upon the veteran's willful misconduct.[6]

Second, if the claimant is found eligible for benefits,[7] the VA then determines whether the veteran qualifies for in-service disability compensation.

Third, if the VA determines that the veteran is entitled to disability compensation, the VA then evaluates the extent of the disability and makes a determination of the percentage of the disability based upon the "Schedule for Rating Disabilities," which is sometimes referred to as the "SRD" and/or the "VASRD."[8] Findings adverse to the interests of the veteran may be appealed administratively.

Fourth, the VA establishes the effective date for the award.

Requirements for Disability Compensation[9]

The purpose of disability compensation is to assist currently disabled veterans whose injury is connected to military service, and to that end, a veteran must meet three basic criteria to the VA's satisfaction:[10]

- *One:* A recent medical diagnosis of a *current* impairment, disability, or disease.
- *Two:* Medical or, on occasion, lay evidence of an *in-service* occurrence or aggravation of the disease or injury.
- *Three:* Medical proof of a *connection* between the current disability and the in-service occurrence or aggravation of an injury or illness.

Each of these requirements is examined below.

Medical Evidence of the Current Impairment or Disability

Disability compensation is available only to veterans with current disabilities.[11] Although a veteran may have been ill or sustained an injury while in service, the mere fact that this occurred is not compensable.

To provide evidence of the current medical problem, the veteran may submit medical records of the current diagnosis and/or treatment. Letters from physicians may be added to the record. Generally speaking, lay evidence of a medical condition is not sufficient. The VA has certain duties to assist veterans in the application process.[12] The VA must assist by providing the veteran with the appropriate records.[13] Usually, the VA is required to provide veterans with a medical exam in order to diagnose a current medical condition.[14] However, in certain circumstances, the VA may not be required to provide such an examination or assistance to the veteran.[15] In addition, the VA must advise veterans of incomplete applications[16] and the evidence needed to evaluate the veteran's claim.[17]

Evidence of an In-Service Occurrence or Aggravation of the Disease or Injury

The second requirement for disability compensation is that there is medical or, under certain circumstances, lay evidence of an in-service occurrence or aggravation of a disease or injury. The in-service requirement is construed broadly. A disability incident or onset of disability is not required to be related to the veteran's military responsibilities and is covered even if it occurred during leave.[18] Further, the evidence submitted on the record must only demonstrate that it is as likely as not that there was an in-service aggravation or occurrence of a disease or injury. When there is nearly equal positive and negative evidence regarding a material issue, the Secretary of Veterans Affairs is required to give the benefit of the doubt to the veteran.[19]

The veteran must submit corroborating evidence of the incident and a statement describing the occurrence, disease, or injury in detail, along with the circumstances surrounding the event.[20] The type of evidence that the veteran must submit may depend upon the type of injury or disease which is being connected to the time of service. For example, a veteran who sustained a fall while in-service might produce evidence of medical treatment for the fall at the time of its occurrence and evidence from military personnel who witnessed the fall.

Medical Proof of a Connection between the In-Service Incident or Aggravation of an Injury/Illness and the Current Disability

This third element requires a *link* between the current injury or illness (requirement 1) and that the disease, injury, or event happened during a period of military service (requirement 2). This requirement is sometimes known as service-connected, the "service connection," or the nexus requirement.

Statutes and regulations require proof of one of five types of connections. *One:* there is a direct connection between the current disability and an incident that happened during the period of military service.[21] *Two:* the current medical condition existed prior to service but was exacerbated during service.[22] *Three:* the current medical problem did not appear during military service, but is presumed to have begun or to be connected with something that occurred during service, either by statute or by VA regulation.[23] *Four:* the present problem is the result of a primary medical condition, and that condition is connected to a period of military service.[24] *Five:* the condition is the result of an injury caused by VA health service, VA training/rehabilitation services, or by participation in a VA sponsored work therapy program.[25]

To establish this connection, the claim must contain adequate medical evidence.[26] What this signifies is that for the in-service connection to be approved, the veteran must have medical proof that the disease, injury, or event which occurred during service *actually caused* the veteran's current disability.

THE VA'S OBLIGATIONS IN THE PREPARATION/PRESENTATION OF THE VETERAN'S CASE AND CERTAIN PRESUMPTIONS

The VA is required by law to use certain standards in reviewing a veteran's claims, and the VA has certain statutory obligations in the preparation of the veteran's case. In addition, statute and regulations provide for certain presumptions of disability as a result of certain occurrences. These standards, requirements, and presumptions are summarized below.

Standard of Proof

As previously explained, in order to receive disability benefits, evidence is required to prove a connection between an in-service incident and a current disability, but in assessing evidence on these elements, the veteran is to be given the "benefit of the doubt."[27] The statute provides that "When there is an approximate balance of positive and negative evidence regarding any issue material to the determination of a matter, the Secretary shall give the benefit of the doubt to the claimant."[28] Regulations provide that when reasonable doubt arises, such doubt will be resolved in favor of the claimant.[29] Hence, in order to satisfy this element, the submitted medical evidence generally needs to show that it is as likely as not that there is a connection between the in-service injury, occurrence, or illness and the current disability.

Assistance in Case Preparation

The VA has a responsibility to assist the veteran in developing a claim. Among other things, the VA is required to advise the veteran of the type of evidence that must be submitted to substantiate the claim.[30]

The VA also must make service and medical records available to veterans for the preparation of their cases.[31] Such records are often crucial in proving the veteran's claim. In many instances, the VA is required to provide veterans with a *medical examination* in order to diagnose the current medical condition.[32] However, under certain circumstances the VA may not be required to provide assistance to the veteran.[33]

Certain Presumptions

In its analysis of certain claims, the VA is required by statute and/or regulation to make certain presumptions.

Presumption of Medical Soundness

In evaluating a veteran's claim, the VA generally presumes that the veteran entered the service in sound medical condition.[34] This may assist the veteran in proving a claim by making it difficult for the VA to claim that the condition or disease existed prior to service. However, if the medical impairment was noted at the time of entry into service, the veteran may have to prove that the condition was exacerbated in-service. If the VA is able to prove by "clear and unmistakable evidence" that the disease or injury was in existence prior to service, and that it was not worsened during service, the veteran's claim will be denied.[35]

Special Rules for Certain In-Service Occurrences

Special rules require the VA to consider a service-connected problem by presumption. For example, certain diseases associated with exposure to Agent Orange will be presumed to be service-related in the case of Vietnam veterans.[36]

A similar regulation holds that veterans who were held prisoners of war or who served in combat can be presumed to have suffered traumatic, stressful events during their military service.[37] Similarly, special rules apply to combat veterans in proving an in-service injury, or other incident.[38] If a combat veteran claims to have suffered a disease, injury, or other event during combat, the VA will usually accept that statement as fact. This is the case even if there are no service records to substantiate the claim.

THE VA RATING SYSTEM

Congress has established by statute a rating system to categorize a veteran's degree of disability for in-service injuries.[39] This system is implemented by the VA through a series of complex regulations and procedures.

After the VA determines that a disability is service-connected, the VA regional office goes through a review process (the "rating activity") to determine the disability rating (on a percentage basis). As used by the VA, the term "disability" is defined as "the average impairment in earning capacity" that results from diseases, injuries, or their resultant aftermath.[40]

Schedule for Rating Disabilities (SRD or VASRD)

By authority of Congress, the VA set up the Schedule for Rating Disabilities ("SRD" or "VASRD"), which rates various disabilities on a percentage basis.[41] The statute provides for 10 grades of disability, and the higher the disability determination, the higher is the monthly compensation that the veteran receives.[42] The VA determines the disability level for an eligible veteran, and Congress sets the compensation rates for veterans based on ratings.[43]

Again, in making individual determinations, the VA and the Board of Veterans' Appeals (BVA) apply the various ratings of the SRD.[44] The SRD is detailed: various sections deal with injuries or diseases that impact particular body functions/parts, including the musculoskeletal system, eyes, and other functions such as hearing, infectious diseases, respiratory system, cardiovascular system, digestive system, genitourinary system, gynecological conditions, and other functions.[45] Each of these sections of the SRD (dealing with a particular body part or function) has a series of medical diagnoses with a numerical diagnostic code (dc) that breaks down percentages of disability based upon the severity of the disability.[46] Each degree of disability under each dc has a description of the symptoms that the claimant veteran must have in order to qualify for that rating. The disability degree increases with the increase in the severity of the symptoms.

Application of the Rating System[47]

Applying this rating system, the VA examines the veteran's medical records to determine the medical diagnosis for the veteran's service-connected disability. The VA then finds the applicable diagnostic code for the disability and finds the degree of disability that is appropriate to the symptoms and diagnosis of the veteran's condition. If a rating falls between two ratings, and the symptoms are closer to the higher rating, then the higher rating will be selected.[48] In makings its determination, the VA examines all of the available evidence, including service records, lay statements, and medical records and other evidence.[49]

Complications in the Use of the Rating System

When the VA applies the diagnostic code(s) to veterans' claims, a number of variables come into play, some of which may be quite complex. And while every rating has unique circumstances, VA ratings in similar cases may not always seem consistent. Having to make fine distinctions within an intricate rating system based on a reading of a veteran's symptoms inevitably leads to some claims that a rating is "wrong" or "underrated."

Another potential complication in the rating process is that a medical condition may be able to be rated under more than one diagnostic code, sometimes to the detriment of the veteran. In addition, not all disabilities and their symptoms and complications are listed on the rating chart, in which case an analogous condition may be used for the rating.[50]

A further complication in the rating system occurs when a veteran has two or more service-connected disabilities. In such a circumstance, the overall percentage of disability is determined by combining the individual ratings, but *not by adding them together.* To calculate the appropriate combined rating, the VA considers each impairment in the order of its severity. Direction on how to make these determinations is contained in the "Combined Rating Table" in the VA regulations.[51]

Changes in Veterans' Ratings

Should the severity of the service-connected disability increase over time, the veteran may apply for an increase in the rated percentage of disability.[52] Similarly, should the condition improve, the ratings percentage may be decreased, and the monthly payments would decrease.

Special Monthly Compensation (SMC)

Veterans with severe disabilities may be entitled to special monthly compensation (SMC) which provides compensation payments at a rate higher than the 100% rate.[53] In addition to the SMC, certain veterans with severe disabilities that require daily assistance or regular health services may be eligible for extra compensation.[54]

Zero Percent Evaluation

If the degree of disability from a service-connected incident does not impair earning capacity, a veteran may receive a 0% rating.[55] However, even a noncompensable evaluation under certain circumstances may entitle the veteran to preferences in federal or state employment and VA health care. A noncompensable evaluation may also be used to document a medical condition if it subsequently worsens.

Periodic Examinations

Following the award of compensation benefits, the VA may require periodic examinations to determine whether the condition is constant in its severity and whether continued payment of disability compensation is warranted.[56] The VA is authorized to reexamine veterans receiving compensation benefits at any time. However, under certain circumstances—for example, if the condition is static—the VA may not schedule review examinations.

Appeals from Ratings

Some veterans may not be satisfied with their disability rating and may wish to appeal the determination. Such an appeal is first undertaken at the local VA level and may eventually proceed to the Court of Veterans Claims ("Court").[57] The Court examines whether the VA considered all of the appropriate facts and set forth a satisfactory explanation for its choice and application of the diagnostic code.

Evaluation of the Rating System

A 2005 Government Accountability Office (GAO) study, *Veterans' Disability Benefits—Claims Processing Challenges and Opportunities for Improvements,*[58] evaluated certain aspects of the disability compensation process. GAO noted that the VA provided $30 billion in cash disability benefits to more than 3.4 million veterans and their survivors in FY2004.[59] GAO found that the VA has continuing challenges in the disability compensation process, including large numbers of pending claims and long processing times.[60]

Another issue that GAO highlighted is the lack of consistency and accuracy of rating decisions at and among the VA's 57 regional offices.[61] Consequently, veterans with similar disabilities may receive different evaluations from the different VA regional offices, and hence may receive significantly different compensation. GAO also noted that the VA's evaluative process has not kept pace with recent developments in medical technology.[62]

GAO uncovered another issue—that more recently discharged veterans with severe injuries would appear to favor a lump sum compensation payment, as opposed to monthly compensation payments over an extended period of time.[63]

RECENT AND PROPOSED LEGISLATION

Veterans' COLA (Cost-of-Living Adjustment)

The veterans' COLA is not automatic. Congress typically has passed legislation annually to provide a COLA in veterans disability compensation equal to the COLA provided under permanent law to recipients of Social Security disability. The Veterans' Compensation Cost-of-Living Adjustment Act of 2008[64] increased, effective December 1, 2008, the rates (dollar amounts) of veterans' disability compensation (and also increased compensation for dependents, the clothing allowance for certain disabled veterans, and the dependency and indemnity compensation for surviving spouses and children).[65]

Similarly, the Veterans' Compensation Cost-of-Living Adjustment Act of 2009[66] increased, effective December 1, 2009, the rates (dollar amounts) of veterans' disability compensation, and also increased compensation for dependents, the clothing allowance for certain disabled veterans, and the dependency and indemnity compensation for surviving spouses and children. The law required that the increase was to be the same percentage as the increase in benefits provided under Title II (Old Age, Survivors, and Disability Insurance) of the Social Security Act, on the same effective date. However, in an unprecedented situation, Congress did not enact a Social Security COLA, so there was no increase for disability compensation benefits, and benefits remained at their 2009 levels (as set by the 2008 legislation).

Legislation has been introduced in the 111th Congress that would create an automatic veterans' COLA based on the Social Security adjustment. S. 3359 (sponsored by Senator John Thune),[67] the proposed Veterans' Disability Compensation Automatic COLA Act, would require that whenever there is an increase in SSI benefits, there would be an increase in veterans' disability benefits by the same percentage amount.

Veterans' Claims Pending and Related Issues

Presently, there is a large number of pending veterans' claims before the VA. According to the VA, which tracks these figures, for the week ended June 5, 2010, there were 546,387 compensation and pension entitlement cases pending.[68] This compares to a pending number of 722,901 rating cases from the time period of June 6, 2009.[69] Concern over this large number of pending claims has been expressed by legislators and veterans' groups.

In response to this large number of pending claims, several bills have been introduced in the 111th Congress that would impact disability determinations by the VA and the manner in which they are processed.

H.R. 3504, the proposed VA Case Backlog Alleviation and Economic Stimulus Act of 2009, was introduced by Representative Jeff Miller.[70] The bill would provide additional funding to the Secretary of Veterans Affairs to hire more claims processors. The bill would require that the Secretary ensure that such processors are assigned proportionately to each state according to the percentage of veterans residing in that state.

H.R. 4121, the proposed Veterans Appeals Improvement and Modernization Act of 2009, was introduced by Representative John J. Hall.[71] The bill provides that if a veteran claimant submits evidence in support of a case for which a substantive appeal has been filed to the Board of Veterans' Appeals, such evidence shall be submitted directly to the Board and not to a regional office of the VA, unless the claimant requests that the evidence first be reviewed by the regional office. The bill would further empower the Court of Appeals for Veterans Claims (CAVC) to affirm, modify, reverse, remand, or vacate and remand a decision of the Board after deciding all relevant assignments of error raised on appeal. Whenever the CAVC reverses a decision on the merits of a particular claim and orders an award of benefits, the CAVC would need not decide any additional assignments of error relating to that claim. The bill would also establish the Veterans Judicial Review Commission to evaluate and make specific decisions to improve the administrative and judicial appellate review processes of veterans' and survivors' benefits determinations.

S. 3286, introduced by Senator Arlen Specter, would require the VA to carry out a pilot program on the award of grants to state and local government agencies and nonprofit organizations to provide assistance to veterans with their submittal of claims to the Veterans Benefits Administration, with the purpose of reducing claim processing time.[72]

S. 3348 was introduced by Senator Daniel K. Akaka.[73] The bill provides that if a claimant adversely affected by a final decision of the Board of Veterans' Appeals who has not filed a notice of appeals with the United States Court of Appeals for Veterans Claims within the required 120-day period files a document with the Board or the agency of original jurisdiction within the 120 days after the Board's decision expressing disagreement with the decision, such document would be treated as a motion for reconsideration by the Board. The bill further provides that such a document would not be considered a motion for reconsideration if the Board or agency of original jurisdiction received the document, determines that it expresses an intent to appeal the decision to the United States Court of Appeals for Veterans Claims, and forwards the document to the CAVC with the 120-day period.

S. 3368 was introduced by Senator Daniel K. Akaka.[74] The bill would authorize the following persons to sign veterans' benefits claims filed on behalf of a person who is under 18, mentally incompetent, or physically unable to sign: (1) a court-appointed representative or person responsible for care; or (2) in the case of an institutionalized person, the manager or principal officer of the institution.

S. 3370 was introduced by Senator Daniel K. Akaka.[75] The bill would amend Title 38 to improve the process by which an individual files jointly for Social Security and dependency and indemnity compensation.

Two companion bills deal with increased disability compensation benefits and related issues. H.R. 1037 was introduced by Representative Stephanie Herseth Sandlin.[76] The companion bill, S. 728, was introduced by Senator Daniel K. Akaka.[77] Among other provisions, the bill would provide increased disability compensation for certain categories of disabled veterans.

End Notes

1 See generally *Federal Benefits for Veterans, Dependents and Survivors*, published by the Departments of Veterans Affairs (2010 edition) (hereinafter cited as "*Federal Benefits*"), available at http://www 1.va.gov/opa/publications/ benefits_book.asp. See CRS Report RL33113, *Veterans Affairs: Basic Eligibility for Disability Benefit Programs*, by Douglas Reid Weimer, regarding the fundamental requirements for disability benefits.

2 *Id.*

3 The severity of the veteran's disability is evaluated by the VA and a determination is made as to what percentage of employment capacity is impaired. See discussion below.

4 See CRS Report RL33113, *Veterans Affairs: Basic Eligibility for Disability Benefit Programs*, by Douglas Reid Weimer, at 2 for a discussion of the disability pension.

5 For further discussion of a disability pension or a non-service-connected pension, see CRS Report RL33113, *Veterans Affairs: Basic Eligibility for Disability Benefit Programs*, at 10-11.

6 See CRS Report RL33113, *Veterans Affairs: Basic Eligibility for Disability Benefit Programs*, at 3-4 in general. For a discussion of "active service" see p. 6, and for a discussion of "willful misconduct" see pp. 8-9.

7 Hence, the claimant becomes a "veteran" for purposes of benefits.

8 38 U.S.C. § 1155; 38 C.F.R. § 4. See discussion below.

9 See Barton F. Stichman et al., *Veterans Benefits Manual* at § 3.1.5. (Hereinafter cited as "*Veterans Benefits Manual*.")

10 For the purposes of this chapter, it is assumed that the claimant/applicant has met the very basic eligibility requirements for VA benefits. The claimant/applicant will be referred to as the "veteran" for the remainder of this chapter.

11 38 U.S.C. §§ 1110, 1131. These provisions deal with the basic entitlement for disability compensation.

12 38 U.S.C. § 5103A.

13 38 U.S.C. §§ 5103A(b),(c).

14 38 U.S.C. § 5103A(d).

[15] 38 U.S.C. § 5103A(a)(2).
[16] 38 U.S.C. § 5102(b).
[17] 38 U.S.C. § 5103(a).
[18] For example, a veteran may receive compensation for a medical condition that resulted from a sports injury incurred during in-service time. See *Veterans Benefit Manual* at §3.1.1.1.
[19] 38 U.S.C. § 5107(b).
[20] 38 C.F.R. § 3.303.
[21] 38 C.F.R. §§ 3.303(a), 3.304, 3.305. See also 38 U.S.C. § 1154. In determining whether the current condition relates to the in-service problem, the VA determines whether the problem is *acute* or *chronic*. An acute problem is considered to be a problem of relatively short duration. A chronic condition is of lengthy duration and may return.
[22] 38 U.S.C. § 1153; 38 C.F.R. § 3.306(a). If the disability existed prior to service, the VA must ascertain whether there was an *increase in the disability during service*. The preexisting problem will not be considered to be aggravated by service if the VA determines that the exacerbation resulted from the natural progression of the disease.
[23] 38 U.S.C. §§ 1112, 1116, 1133; 38 C.F.R. §§ 3.307-3.309; 38 C.F.R. § 3.313(b). If the disability claimed is a disease which was not diagnosed or recorded on the veteran's service record, the VA is required to ascertain whether the *incubation time* for the disease could have started during in-service time (38 C.F.R. § 3.03(d)).
[24] 38 C.F.R. § 3.310(a). If the disability claimed cannot be determined to be in-service, either directly or by exacerbation, the VA will then decide whether the problem may be *service-connected on a secondary basis*. This reasoning is based on the theory that it was proximately caused by a service-connected condition. For instance, a primary disease is contracted in service. A related, secondary disease develops as a result of the primary disease.
[25] 38 U.S.C. § 1151.
[26] 38 U.S.C. § 5107.
[27] 38 U.S.C. § 5107(b).
[28] *Id.*
[29] 38 C.F.R. § 3.102.
[30] 38 U.S.C. § 5103(a).
[31] 38 U.S.C. §§ 5103A(b)(c).
[32] 38 U.S.C. § 5103A(d).
[33] 38 U.S.C. § 5103A(a)(2).
[34] 38 U.S.C. § 1111.
[35] *Id.*
[36] 38 C.F.R. § 3.307(a)(6)(iii). See generally, CRS Report RL34370, *Veterans Affairs: Health Care and Benefits for Veterans Exposed to Agent Orange*, by Sidath Viranga Panangala and Douglas Reid Weimer.
[37] 38 C.F.R. § 3.304(f).
[38] 38 U.S.C. § 1154(b); 38 C.F.R. § 3.304(d)(f).
[39] 38 U.S.C. § 1155.
[40] 38 C.F.R. § 4.1.
[41] 38 U.S.C. § 1155.
[42] 10% through 100%.
[43] The current monthly rates, effective on December 1, 2008, are as follows: An unmarried veteran without dependents and with a 10% disability receives $123 per month. The rates increase to a 100% disability payment of $2,673 per month (for an unmarried veteran without dependents). For rate tables and a compensation calculator, see http://www.vba.va.gov/bln/21/rates/comp0108.htm. *The payment rates are not automatically adjusted for inflation, and are only increased if Congress passes enabling legislation.* Congress usually grants an increase based on the consumer price index or the cost-of-living formula used to determine the Social Security old age increase. The 2009 rates were set by P.L. 110-324, 110th Cong., 2d Sess. (September 24, 2008), the Veterans' Compensation Cost-of-Living Adjustment Act of 2008. As discussed below, P.L. 111-37, 111th Cong., 1st Sess. (June 30, 2009), the Veterans' Compensation Cost-of-Living Adjustment Act of 2009, provided for an increase in disability benefits equal to the increase provided for Social Security benefits. In an unprecedented situation, in 2009, Congress did not enact a COLA for 2010 Social Security Benefits. The practical effect of this situation is that although an increase for disability benefits was enacted, the monthly benefits remain at their 2009 levels (as enacted in 2008).
[44] 38 C.F.R. § 4.1.
[45] For example see 38 C.F.R. §§ 4.40 to 4.73 for the musculoskeletal system; 38 C.F.R. §§ 4.75 to 4.84a for the eyes.
[46] See 38 C.F.R. § 4.84a for an example of the ratings and diagnostic codes chart for impairment of vision.
[47] See CRS Report RL33991, *Disability Evaluation of Military Servicemembers*, by Christine Scott and Don J. Jansen.
[48] 38 C.F.R. § 4.7.

[49] 38 C.F.R. § 3.103(d).
[50] 38 C.F.R. § 4.20. However, if a veteran's disability is so extraordinary or unusual that an analogy cannot be made through use of the rating charts, an "extraschedular rating" for a veteran may be made (38 C.F.R. § 3.321(b)).
[51] 38 U.S.C. § 1157; 38 C.F.R. § 4.25.
[52] See "Compensation and Pension Service" section at VA website; *A Summary of VA Benefits: Putting Veterans First*, VA Pamphlet 21-00-1 (April 2008); see also http://www.va.gov (click on "Veteran Services"; then go to "General Benefits Information"; then go to "Compensation and Pension").
[53] 38 U.S.C. § 1114(k); 38 C.F.R. § 3.350. Such disabilities may involve the loss of use of a hand or foot and other serious impairments.
[54] 38 U.S.C. § 1114(r)(2); 38 C.F.R. § 3.352.
[55] Many conditions listed within the ratings tables are rated as 0. See also 38 C.F.R. § 4.31.
[56] 38 C.F.R. § 3.327(a).
[57] See CRS Report RS22561, *Veterans Affairs: The U.S. Court of Appeals for Veterans Claims—Judicial Review of VA Decision Making*, by Douglas Reid Weimer.
[58] GAO-06-283T, Testimony before the Committee on Veterans' Affairs, House of Representatives; Statement for the Record by Cynthia A. Bascetta, Director, Education, Workforce, and Income Security Issues (GAO) (December 7, 2005).
[59] *Id.* at 1.
[60] *Id.* at 2, 4-6.
[61] *Id.* at 5-7.
[62] *Id.* at 8-9.
[63] *Id.* at 9-10.
[64] P.L. 110-430, 110th Cong., 2d Sess. (September 24, 2008).
[65] This law amended 38 U.S.C. § 1114 and established increased monthly payments.
[66] P.L. 111-37, 111th Cong., 1st Sess. (June 30, 2009).
[67] S. 3359, 111th Cong., 2d Sess. (2010). The bill was introduced and referred to the Senate Committee on Veterans' Affairs on May 13, 2010.
[68] The VA breaks these figures down in very detailed "workload reports." For more information, go to the VA website, http://www.va.gov, and search under "workload reports." Then go to "2010 Monday Morning Workload Report" and access for the current statistics.
[69] *Id.*
[70] H.R. 3504, 111th Cong., 1st Sess. (2009). The bill was introduced and referred to the House Appropriations Committee and the House Veterans' Affairs Committee on July 31, 2009.
[71] H.R. 4121, 111th Cong., 1st Sess. (2009). The bill was introduced and referred to the House Committee on Veterans' Affairs on November 19, 2009, and was referred to the House Subcommittee on Disability Assistance and Memorial Affairs on November 20, 2009.
[72] S. 3286, 111th Cong., 2d Sess. (2010). The bill was introduced and referred to the Senate Committee on Veterans' Affairs on April 29, 2010. The committee held hearings on May 19, 2010.
[73] S. 3348, 111th Cong., 2d Sess. (2010). The bill was introduced and referred to the Senate Committee on Veterans' Affairs on May 12, 2010. The committee held hearings on May 19, 2010.
[74] S. 3368, 111th Cong., 2d Sess. (2010). The bill was introduced and referred to the Senate Committee on Veterans' Affairs on May 13, 2010. The committee held hearings on May 19, 2010.
[75] S. 3370, 111th Cong., 2d Sess. (2010). The bill was introduced and referred to the Senate Committee on Veterans' Affairs on May 13, 2010. The committee held hearings on May 19, 2010.
[76] H.R. 1037, 111th Cong., 1st Sess. (2009). The bill was introduced in the House on February 12, 2009, and passed the House on July 14, 2009. It passed the Senate on October 7, 2009. A message on the Senate action was sent to the House on October 8, 2009.
[77] S. 728, 111th Cong., 1st Sess. (2009). The bill was introduced in the Senate on March 26, 2009, and the Senate passed the companion measure, H.R. 1037, on October 7, 2009.

In: Veterans Benefits
Editors: George B. Meyers and Alice M. Glaskin ISBN: 978-1-61209-581-3

Chapter 4

VETERANS' BENEFITS: BENEFITS AVAILABLE FOR DISABLED VETERANS

Christine Scott and Carol D. David

SUMMARY

Although U.S. Armed Forces are deployed around the globe, a number of servicemembers are currently serving in the Operation Enduring Freedom (OEF) and Operation Iraq Freedom (OIF) combat zones. As a result of the risks facing these servicemembers, some of them are incurring injuries or illnesses during their active service (or having existing medical conditions worsen as a result of their service). Congress has shown an interest in the treatment of injured servicemembers while undergoing medical treatment and their transition from military to civilian life as veterans. An injured servicemember (or veteran) may require specific types of assistance or benefits to enable him or her to have a better quality of life.

The Department of Veterans Affairs (VA) provides a range of benefits for veterans. However, certain benefits have specifically been created to assist disabled veterans.

Disability compensation provides a monthly cash benefit to veterans whose disabilities resulted from injury or disease contracted in or aggravated by military service. The amount is based on the level of disability.

The Vocational Rehabilitation and Employment (VR&E) program is designed to help veterans with service-connected disabilities prepare for, find, and keep suitable jobs. Assistance is also available to help veterans with living skills.

Automobile and special adaptive equipment grants are available to certain disabled veterans and servicemembers to purchase new or used automobiles (or other conveyances) to accommodate a disability.

Clothing allowances are designed for certain veterans entitled to receive compensation for a service-connected disability for which he or she uses a prosthetic or orthopedic device.

Housing grants are provided for constructing an adapted home or modifying an existing home to meet the adaptive needs of certain veterans and servicemembers. There are three grant programs available for permanent residences, and two of the three grant programs are also available for temporary residences.

Service Disabled Veterans' Insurance (S-DVI) is life insurance for veterans who have received a service-connected disability rating by the VA.

This chapter provides information on these benefits, including eligibility, history, and the application process. Information regarding spending and the beneficiaries of these benefits is in the **Appendix** to this chapter.

Although U.S. Armed Forces are deployed around the globe, a number of servicemembers are currently serving in the Operation Enduring Freedom (OEF) and Operation Iraq Freedom (OIF) combat zones. As a result of the risks facing these servicemembers, some of them are incurring injuries or illnesses during their active service (or having existing medical conditions worsen as a result of their service). Congress has shown an interest in the treatment of injured servicemembers while undergoing medical treatment and their transition from military to civilian life as veterans. An injured servicemember (or veteran) may require specific types of assistance or benefits to enable him or her to have a better quality of life.

The VA provides a range of benefits for veterans who meet certain eligibility criteria. However, certain benefits have specifically been created to assist disabled veterans. Among them are disability compensation, the vocational rehabilitation and employment program, automobile and special adaptive equipment grants, clothing allowances grants, adapted housing grants, and service-disabled veterans' insurance.

This chapter provides information on these benefits, including eligibility, legislative history, and the application process. The **Appendix** provides a table with the number of beneficiaries and FY2009 outlays (spending) for each of the benefits discussed in this chapter.

DISABILITY COMPENSATION

Disability compensation provides a monthly cash benefit to veterans who have incurred an injury or disease contracted in, or aggravated by, active military service.[1] The benefit level is determined by the level of disability.[2] A disability rating is assigned (from 0% to 100% in increments of 10%) by the VA after a physical examination of all body systems for which the veteran is claiming a disability. However, a cash benefit is only provided to veterans with a rating of 10% or more.

The basic benefit amount ranges from $123 to $2,673 per month, depending on the disability rating. Additional amounts can be paid in certain circumstances, including severe disabilities or loss of limbs; having a spouse, dependent children,[3] or dependent parents; or having a disabled spouse.

Legislative History

Prior to World War I, disability compensation was a component of the pension program based on military service in a particular conflict. The World War Veterans Act of 1924 (P.L.

242), later codified by P.L. 85-56 and P.L 85-857, established the modern disability compensation program.[4]

Eligibility and Application Process

A veteran may be eligible for disability compensation if (1) the veteran is disabled resulting from personal injury suffered or disease contracted in the line of duty, or for aggravation of a preexisting injury suffered or disease contracted in the line of duty, in the active military, naval, or air service, during a period of war and (2) if the veteran was discharged or released under conditions other than dishonorable from the period of service in which the injury was incurred.[5] The VA makes a case-by-case determination of whether the discharge was under "conditions other than dishonorable" and can review dishonorable discharges to determine whether the veteran may be eligible for VA benefits.[6]

The application process requires proving a medical diagnosis of current disability, medical evidence of the in-service incident or the worsening of an injury or disease, and a link between the in-service incident or the worsening of a disease and military service. To apply, a veteran completes VA Form 2 1-526 and provides the following materials: discharge or separation papers (Department of Defense Form DD214 or its equivalent) and dependency records (marriage license and children's birth certificates). The VA will then review the documentation and schedule an examination for the disability evaluation.

After the examination, a disability rating is assigned. If the rating is 10% or more, the veteran will then receive his or her disability compensation payment at the beginning of the next month.

Vocational Rehabilitation and Employment Program

The Vocational Rehabilitation and Employment (VR&E) program is designed to help veterans with service-connected disabilities prepare for, find, and keep suitable jobs. Veterans with severe service-connected disabilities who cannot immediately consider work are offered other services by the VR&E to improve their ability to live as independently as possible.[7]

Legislative History

The vocational rehabilitation program for veterans began in 1918. With the end of World War I, concerns were raised about ensuring that returning disabled servicemembers be provided a mechanism for resuming productive economic lives. The Vocational Rehabilitation Act (P.L. 65- 178), which was enacted by Congress in 1918, provided for "vocational rehabilitation and return to civil employment of disabled persons discharged from military or naval forces of the United States."[8]

Under current law, the VR&E program must provide a number of services including the following:[9]

- a comprehensive rehabilitation evaluation to determine a veteran's abilities, skills, interests, and needs;
- vocational counseling and rehabilitation planning;
- employment services such as job-seeking skills, resumé development, and other work readiness assistance;
- assistance finding and keeping a job (including the use of special employer incentives);
- on-the-job training, apprenticeships, and non-paid work experiences (if needed);
- post-secondary training at a college, vocational, technical, or business school;
- supportive rehabilitation services (including case management, counseling, and referral); and
- independent living services.

Eligibility and entitlement must be established for participation in this program. A veteran who has an employment handicap and is eligible for the VR&E program is entitled to all applicable services.

Eligibility and Application Process

The eligibility process involves a two-step process to establish eligibility and entitlement. To be eligible in the VR&E program, a veteran must (1) have received or will receive a discharge that is other than dishonorable and (2) have a service-connected disability rating of at least 10%.[10]

There is a limitation in the period of eligibility. VR&E services may be used up to 12 years from the latter of the following dates:

- date of separation from active military service or
- date the veteran was first notified by the VA of a service-connected disability rating.

The period of eligibility may be extended if a Vocational Rehabilitation Counselor (VRC) determines that a veteran has a serious employment handicap.

After eligibility is established, the veteran meets with a VRC for a comprehensive evaluation to determine whether the veteran is entitled to services. The comprehensive evaluation includes the following:

- an assessment of the veteran's interests, aptitudes, and abilities;
- an assessment of whether service-connected disabilities impair the veteran's ability to find or hold a job using the occupational skills that he or she has already developed; and
- vocational exploration and goal development.

An entitlement determination is required to enter the VR&E program. On the basis of the results of the comprehensive evaluation, a VRC determines whether a veteran has an employment handicap. A veteran is entitled to services if the veteran is within the period of eligibility, has a 20% or greater service-connected disability rating, and has an employment handicap.

If the service-connected disability rating is less than 20% or if the veteran is beyond the period of eligibility, then a serious employment handicap must be found to establish entitlement to VR&E services.

After the entitlement determination is made, the VRC and the veteran work together to

- select a VR&E program track leading to an employment or independent living goal;
- identify viable employment or independent living service options;
- determine transferable skills;
- explore labor market and wage information;
- identify physical demands and other job characteristics;
- narrow vocational options to identify a suitable employment goal;
- investigate training requirements;
- identify resources needed to achieve rehabilitation; and
- develop an individualized rehabilitation plan to achieve the identified employment or independent living goal.

The rehabilitation plan is an individualized written outline of the services, resources, and criteria that will be used to achieve successful rehabilitation. It is an agreement that is signed by the veteran and the VRC and is reviewed annually to determine whether any changes are needed.

Depending on their circumstances, veterans will work with their VRCs to select one of the following five tracks of services:[11]

- re-employment;
- rapid employment services for new employment;
- self-employment;
- employment through long-term services; or
- independent living services.

After a rehabilitation plan is developed and signed, a VRC or case manager will continue to work with the veteran to implement the plan to achieve suitable employment or independent living. The VRC or case manager may coordinate services such as tutorial assistance, training in job-seeking skills, medical and dental referrals, adjustment counseling, payment of training allowance, if applicable, and other services as required to achieve rehabilitation.

If a veteran is found to be ineligible for services, the VRC will help him or her locate other resources to address any rehabilitation and employment needs identified during the evaluation. Other resources that the veteran may be referred to include state vocational rehabilitation programs, Department of Labor employment programs for disabled veterans, local agencies providing services for employment or small business development, Internet-based resources for rehabilitation and employment, and information about applying for financial aid.

AUTOMOBILE AND SPECIAL ADAPTIVE EQUIPMENT GRANTS

Financial assistance is available to certain disabled veterans and servicemembers to purchase new or used automobiles (or other conveyances) to accommodate a disability. The veteran or servicemember may only receive the automobile grant once in his or her lifetime. The grant is up to $11,000 ($18,000 beginning October 1, 2011) and is paid directly to the seller of the automobile to be applied to the total price of the automobile.[12] Certain veterans who need to have a vehicle specially adapted due to their service-connected disability may qualify for the adaptive equipment grant.

Legislative History

P.L. 79-663 in 1946 and P.L. 80-785 in 1948 appropriated funding for helping disabled World War II veterans in purchasing automobiles. The two laws specified a $1,600 per-vehicle allowance, but they did not place a limitation on the number of cars a veteran could purchase. Because this limitation was not in place, some qualified veterans could not receive benefits due to a shortfall in funding.

In 1950, P.L. 81-798 authorized the VA to pay up to $1,600 of the costs for disabled World War II veterans to purchase specially adapted automobiles, with a limit of one assisted automobile purchase per veteran. The benefit amount has increased over the years. Most recently, The Transportation Equity Act of the 21st Century (P.L. 105-178) increased the benefit amount from $5,500 to $8,000; the Veterans Education and Benefits Expansion Act of 2001 (P.L. 107-103) increased the benefit amount to $9,000; and the Veterans Benefits Act of 2003 (P.L. 108-183) increased the benefit amount to $11,000. The Veterans' Benefits Act of 2010 (P.L. 111-275) increased the benefit amount to $18,000 effective October 2, 1011, and provided for an annual inflation adjustment to this amount.

Eligibility and Application Process

The adapted automobile grants are available to any veteran or servicemember entitled to compensation as the result of certain injuries incurred or diseases contracted in or aggravated by active military, naval, or air service. Those specific injuries include the loss or permanent loss of use of one or both feet, one or both hands, or permanent impairment of vision.[13] The Veterans' Benefits Act of 2010 (P.L. 111-275) expanded eligibility to include veterans with a severe burn injury effective October 2, 2011.

Veterans can apply for the grant by submitting VA Form 21-4502 (completing only Section I) to the local VA regional office to establish entitlement. The VA will complete Section II, which certifies eligibility, and return the original to the veteran. The veteran is then responsible for obtaining the invoice from the seller, completing Section III, and submitting the completed form to the local VA regional office.

If the veteran is entitled to adaptive equipment only (i.e., service-connected for ankylosis, or stiff or fixed joints, of the knees or hips), the veteran would complete VA Form 10-1394, *Application for Adaptive Equipment-Motor Vehicle,* and submit it to the local VA medical center. Additionally, VA Form 10-1394 should be completed for approval of equipment not specified on VA Form 21- 4502.

Clothing Allowance Grant

The clothing allowance benefit is designed for any veteran who is entitled to receive compensation for a service-connected disability for which he or she uses a prosthetic or orthopedic device. The allowance is also available to any veteran whose service-connected skin condition requires prescribed medication that irreparably damages the veteran's outer garments.

Legislative History

In 1972, Congress mandated under P.L. 92-3 28 that the VA Administrator shall pay a clothing allowance to each veteran because of a service-connected disability. This law was passed due to disability devices wearing out or tearing up the clothing of the veteran. The allowance was originally set at $150 per year, but it has been increased by legislation to the current annual level of $677.[14]

Eligibility and Application Process

To apply for the annual clothing allowance, a veteran completes VA Form 10-8678.[15]

Enrollment for the benefit is for one year. Each year the enrollment is reviewed and may be renewed depending upon the priority group.[16] Priority groups range from 1 to 8 with 1 being the highest priority for enrollment. This assignment is based on eligibility status, which is determined during the application process.[17]

Adapted Housing Grants

Housing grants are provided for constructing an adapted home or modifying an existing home to meet the adaptive needs of veterans and totally disabled members of the Armed Forces before discharge or release from the Armed Forces. There are three major grant programs:

- The Specially Adapted Housing (SAH) grant, available for permanent and some temporary residences, which is focused on the construction or acquisition of a specially adapted home, or remodeling of an existing home into a specially adapted home for veterans and servicemembers;
- The Special Home Adaptation (SHA) grant, available for permanent and some temporary residences, which is focused on adapting homes to reduce the barriers to living for veterans and servicemembers; and

- The Home Improvements and Structural Alterations (HISA) grant, available for permanent residences, which is focused on improvements necessary for treatment continuation, or for disability access to the home and essential lavatory and sanitary facilities for disabled veterans.

Specially Adapted Housing Grant

The SAH grants are focused on the construction or acquisition of a specially adapted home, or remodeling of an existing home into a specially adapted home for veterans and servicemembers. The goal is to provide a barrier-free living environment that affords the veteran or servicemember a level of independent living that he or she may not have otherwise enjoyed. The grant is currently limited to $60,000 per lifetime, and it may be used up to three times. [18]

The VA can provide an SAH grant of up to $14,000 to disabled veterans and servicemembers temporarily living in a home owned by a family member. This program for temporary residence grants is scheduled to expire on December 31, 2011.[19]

Eligibility

The SAH benefit is available to veterans and servicemembers who have service-connected disabilities. These service-connected disabilities entitles them to compensation for permanent and total disability due to

- the loss or loss of use of both lower extremities, such as to prevent movement without the aid of braces, crutches, canes, or a wheelchair;
- blindness in both eyes, having only light perception, plus the loss of use of one lower extremity;
- the loss or loss of use of one lower extremity together with (1) residual of organic disease or injury, or (2) the loss or loss of use of one upper extremity, which also affects the functions of balance or propulsion so as to prevent movement without the aid of braces, crutches, canes, or a wheelchair;
- disability due to a severe burn injury; and
- the loss or loss of use of both upper extremities such as to prevent the use of the arms at or above the elbow.

In addition, it must be medically feasible for the veteran or servicemember to live in the house; the house must be adapted to meet the veteran's or servicemember's needs; and it must be feasible, with the grant assistance, for the veteran or servicemember to buy the house.

Application Process

To apply for the SAH grant, a veteran or servicemember completes and submits VA Form 26- 4555, *Veterans Application in Acquiring Specially Adapted Housing or Special Home Adaptation Grant*, to the local VA regional office.

Special Home Adaptation Grant

The VA also offers the SHA grant. This grant is used to assist disabled veterans and servicemembers with mobility throughout their homes. The grant is currently limited to $12,000 per lifetime, and it may be used up to three times.

The VA can provide an SHA grant of up to $2,000 to disabled veterans and servicemembers temporarily living in a home owned by a family member. This program for temporary residence grants is scheduled to expire on December 31, 2011.[20]

Eligibility

The SHA grant is available to veterans and servicemembers who have service-connected disabilities, entitling them to compensation for permanent and total disability due to

- blindness in both eyes with 5/200 visual acuity or less;
- the anatomical loss or loss of use of both hands or extremities below the elbow; or
- a severe burn injury.

Application Process

To apply for the SHA grant, a veteran or servicemember completes and submits VA Form 26-4555, *Veterans Application in Acquiring Specially Adapted Housing or Special Home Adaptation Grant*, to the local VA regional office.

Home Improvements and Structural Alterations Grant

Under the HISA grant program, assistance is provided for any home improvement necessary for the continuation of the disabled veteran's treatment, or for disability access to the home and essential lavatory and sanitary facilities. A HISA grant is available to veterans who have received medical determinations indicating that improvements and structural alterations are necessary or appropriate for the effective and economical treatment of their disabilities. A veteran may receive both a HISA grant and either an SHA or SAH grant.

Eligibility

The HISA program is available for both service-connected disabled veterans and non service- connected disabled veterans as detailed below:

- home improvement benefits up to $4,100 may be provided to service-connected disabled veterans; and
- home improvement benefits up to $1,200 may be provided to nonserviceconnected disabled veterans.

Application Process

To apply for the HISA grant, the veteran completes and submits VA Form 10-0103, *Veterans Application for Assistance in Acquiring Home Improvement and Structural Alterations* to the local VA medical center.[21]

Legislative History of Adapted Housing Benefits

In 1948, P.L. 80-702 authorized the VA to pay up to 50% of the cost for a disabled veteran to purchase a new home or modify existing housing to adapt it to accommodate his or her disability. The law had a one-year limitation (after discharge) for the entitlement, but this was flexible under specific circumstances. It also gave the VA authority to add other chronic diseases within its eligibility lists.

In 2006, the Veterans' Housing Opportunity and Benefits Improvement Act (P.L. 109-233) permitted the use of SHA and SAH grants for temporary residences and made several significant changes to the SAH benefit. An eligible veteran or active duty servicemember can now use the benefit for up to three occurrences as long as the aggregate granted by the administrator does not exceed the maximum amount allowable.

The Housing and Economic Recovery Act of 2008 (P.L. 110-289) made several changes related to home modifications for veterans:

- amended eligibility Chapter 21 of Title 38, United States Code, by inserting after Section 2101 that members of the Armed Forces with service-connected disabilities and individuals residing outside the United States are also eligible for adapted housing benefits and assistance;
- added assistance for members of the Armed Forces with service-connected disabilities residing temporarily in housing owned by a family member;
- amended Section 2101 of Title 38, United States Code, by providing specially
- adapted housing assistance for individuals with severe burn injuries;
- amended Section 21 02A(e) of Title 38, United States Code, by extending assistance for individuals residing temporarily in housing owned by a family member; and
- increased the benefit amount for specially adapted housing for disabled veterans.

The Veterans' Benefits Improvement Act of 2008 (P.L. 110-389) required the Secretary to provide, at no cost, a handbook to veterans of appropriate designs for specially adapted housing. The handbook is to be updated every six years to take into account new or unique disabilities.

SERVICE DISABLED VETERANS' INSURANCE

Service Disabled Veterans' Insurance (S-DVI) is life insurance for veterans who have received a service-connected disability rating from the VA. The basic S-DVI program insures eligible veterans for up to $10,000 of coverage. Veterans who have basic S-DVI coverage and are totally disabled before age 65 are eligible to have their premiums waived.[22]

If a premium waiver is granted, a totally disabled veteran may apply for additional coverage up to $20,000 ($30,000 beginning October 1, 2011) under the Supplemental S-DVI program. Premiums for Supplemental S-DVI coverage, however, cannot be waived. The cost varies depending upon age, type of plan, and the amount of coverage.[23]

Legislative History

The Insurance Act of 1951 (P.L. 85-857) established the Service-Disabled Veterans' Insurance (S-DVI) program for veterans with service-connected disabilities. S-DVI is open to veterans who separated from the service on or after April 25, 1951, who received a service-connected disability rating of 0% or greater. The Veterans' Benefit Act of 1992 (P.L. 102-568) adjusted the current program and provided for $20,000 of supplemental coverage to S-DVI policyholders.[24]

To protect veterans who become incompetent from a service-connected disability while eligible to apply for S-DVI and who die before an application is filed, P.L 85-857 was amended in 1991 by P.L. 102-86. This insurance is issued posthumously, and it is payable to a preferred class of the veteran's relatives in a lump sum.[25]

To provide veterans with financial relief from high premium rates at advanced ages, S-DVI term premiums were "capped" at the age 70 renewal rate effective November 1, 2000, by P.L. 106-419. This means that the annual premium for these policies will not exceed $69.73 per $1,000 of coverage.

The Veterans' Benefits Improvements Act of 2008 (P.L. 110-389) provided that the costs of administering the insurance program be paid from premiums credited to the fund, and that payments for claims in excess of premiums credited (after administrative expenses are paid) are to be paid from appropriations.

The Veterans' Benefits Act of 2010 (P.L. 111-275) increased the maximum amount of supplemental coverage to $30,000 effective October 1, 2011.

Eligibility and Application Process

To be eligible for S-DVI, a veteran must have[26]

- received other than a dishonorable discharge;
- been released from active duty after April 25, 1951; and
- received a rating for a new service-connected disability within the last two years.

However, the veteran does not need to have a 100% rating to be eligible. Veterans who receive a new rating of even 0% are eligible for the coverage.[27] The veteran must apply for the insurance within two years from the date he or she is notified that service-connection has been established.

S-DVI policyholders are eligible for supplemental coverage if

- they are eligible for a waiver of premiums on their S-DVI policy due to total disability;
- they apply for the coverage within one year from notice of the grant of waiver; or
- they are under the age of 65.

A veteran applies for the basic S-DVI using the VA Form 29-43 64. To apply for the supplemental S-DVI, the veteran must complete VA Form 29-0189 or submit a letter requesting supplemental S-DVI. To receive a total disability waiver of S-DVI premiums, a veteran must fill out VA Form 29-357. Submission of all forms can be done at the local VA regional office or online at the VA website.[28]

APPENDIX. UTILIZATION OF BENEFITS FOR DISABLED VETERANS

Table A-1. Beneficiaries and Spending on Benefits for Disabled Veterans in FY2009

Benefit	Number of Beneficiaries (in thousands)	Outlays (Spending) (in millions of $)
Disability Compensation(for veterans)	3,014.7	35,413.7
Vocational Rehabilitation and Education (for veterans, spouses, and certain dependents)[a]	72.8	612.5
Adaptive Automobile and Equipment Grants (for disabled veterans and servicemembers)	8.6	56.0
Clothing Allowances (for veterans)	97.8	68.5
Specially Adapted Housing Grant (for veterans and disabled servicemembers)	1.3	56.7
Service Disabled Veterans' Insurance(for veterans)[b]	174.4	105.7

Source. Table provided by the CRS compilation of data from the Department of Veteran Affairs (VA), *FY2010 Budget Submission Benefits and Burial Programs and Departmental Administration,* Volume 3 of 4, Table, pp. 2A-2 to 2A-3, 2B-2 to 2B-3, and 2G-10 to 2G11. Available at http://www.va.gov/budget/summary/2010/Volume_3- Benefits_and_Burial_and_Dept_Admin.pdf.

a. This does not include those receiving VR&E counseling services.

b. Outlays for Service-Disabled Veterans' Insurance are gross outlays.

End Notes

[1] 38 U.S.C. § 1131.

[2] For more information on the VA's disability rating schedule, see CRS Report RL33991, *Disability Evaluation of Military Servicemembers*, Disability Evaluation of Military Servicemembers, by Christine Scott, Sidath Viranga Panangala, and Charles A. Henning; and for a more thorough description of the rating process, see CRS Report RL33323, *Veterans Affairs: Benefits for Service-Connected Disabilities*, by Douglas Reid Weimer.

[3] This includes children between the ages of 18 and 23 attending college.

[4] For more information on the legislative history of the disability compensation program, see *VA Disability Compensation Program Legislative History December 2004 Report,* by VA Office of Policy, Planning, and Preparedness, pp. 33-39, available at *Compensation Program Legislative History December 2004 Report*).

[5] 38 U.S.C. § 1110.

[6] For a more detailed description of eligibility and the claims process, see CRS Report RL33 113, *Veterans Affairs: Basic Eligibility for Disability Benefit Programs*, by Douglas Reid Weimer.

[7] 38 U.S.C. § 3102.

[8] *VA Disability Compensation Program Legislative History December 2004 Report.*

[9] For more information regarding the services of the VR&E program, see CRS Report RL34627, *Veterans' Benefits: The Vocational Rehabilitation and Employment Program*, by Christine Scott and Carol D. Davis.

[10] 38 U.S.C. § 3102.

[11] For more information on the five tracks of services, see CRS Report RL34627, *Veterans' Benefits: The Vocational Rehabilitation and Employment Program*, by Christine Scott and Carol D. Davis.

[12] 38 U.S.C. § 3902.

[13] 38 U.S.C. § 3901.
[14] 38 U.S.C. § 1162. The current level of $677 was payable beginning on August 1, 2008.
[15]To download this form, go to https://www.1010ez.med.va.gov/sec/vha/1010ez/.
[16] For more information regarding this benefit, contact the nearest VA Regional Office.
[17] For more information on priority group assignment, see CRS Report RL33993, *Veterans' Health Care Issues*, by Sidath Viranga Panangala.
[18] 38 U.S.C. § 2101.
[19] For more information on active duty adaptive housing grants, see http://www.homeloans.va.gov/sah.htm.
[20] For more information on active duty adaptive housing grants, see http://www.homeloans.va.gov/sah.htm.
[21] For more information, see http://www.homeloans.va.gov/sah.htm.
[22] 38 U.S.C. § 1922.
[23] For more information on S-DVI see CRS Report R41435, *Veterans' Benefits: Current Life Insurance Programs* , by Christine Scott.
[24] Ibid.
[25] For a definition of the preferred class of veteran's relatives, see *VA Life Insurance Programs for Veterans and Servicemembers 2008 Booklet,* at http://www.insurance.va.gov/inForceGliSite/GLIhandbook/glibooklet.pdf.
[26] 38 U.S.C. § 1922.
[27] A veteran can have a service-connected disability with a rating of 0%.
[28] For more information on the veteran's insurance application process, refer to http://www.insurance.va.gov/inForceGliSite/buying/SDVI.htm.

In: Veterans Benefits
Editors: George B. Meyers and Alice M. Glaskin
ISBN: 978-1-61209-581-3

Chapter 5

VETERANS HEALTH CARE: PROJECT HERO IMPLEMENTATION

Sidath Viranga Panangala

SUMMARY

In general, the Department of Veterans Affairs (VA), through the Veterans Health Administration (VHA), provides a majority of medical services to veterans within its health care system. However, in some instances, such as when a clinical service cannot be provided by a VA medical center, when a veteran is unable to access VA health care facilities due to geographic inaccessibility, or in emergencies when delays could lead to life threatening situations, VHA is authorized by law to send the veteran outside of VA's health care system to seek care. In 2006, the conference report to accompany the Military Quality of Life and Veterans Affairs Appropriations Act of 2006 (P.L. 109-114, H.Rept. 109-305) directed the VA to implement a cost-effective purchased care management program and to develop at least three pilot programs to encourage collaboration with industry and academia. In response to this requirement, VHA established a demonstration program to enhance the existing fee basis care program that was named Project HERO (Healthcare Effectiveness through Resource Optimization).

In October 2007, VA awarded a contract to Humana Veterans Healthcare Services (HVHS) for medical/surgical, mental health, diagnostic and dialysis services, and the contract became operational in January 2008. Under Project HERO, HVHS maintains a prescreened network of health care providers who meet VA quality standards.

In general, when a patient requires a specific service, and the local VA medical center does not have the specific medical expertise or the technologies to meet that necessity, the local VA medical center authorizes the specific service to be provided under Project HERO. Once the veteran receives care, HVHS is contractually required to return the patient's medical record to the local VA medical center, and HVHS sends the claims data to VA for reimbursement.

VHA's contract and fee basis care expenditures are of interest to Congress for at least two reasons. First, expenditures for contract and fee basis care services are increasing, and second, concerns have been raised about the fee basis care program. Specifically, VA's Office of Inspector General (OIG) has reported that VHA has made a significant number of improper payments for fee basis care as well as in some instances has not properly justified and authorized fee basis care. Given these concerns, and the establishment of the Project HERO demonstration as a means to better manage non-VA provided care, at least two broad policy questions may be of interest to Congress: (1) Has Project HERO enhanced the existing fee basis care program? and (2) Are there lessons to be learned from the Project HERO demonstration that could be applied to standardize the fee basis care program throughout the VA health care system?

This chapter first provides a brief overview of the VA health care system, followed by a overview of Project HERO. Second, it discuses the current fee basis care process, as well as the implementation of Project HERO. The report concludes with a discussion of observations on the implementation of Project HERO based on VHA and HVHS perspectives. It should be noted that although dental care services are a component of Project HERO, and are provided through Dental Federal Services (Delta Dental), this chapter does not discuss dental care services provided under Project HERO.

INTRODUCTION AND OVERVIEW OF THE VA HEALTH CARE SYSTEM

The Department of Veterans Affairs (VA), through the Veterans Health Administration (VHA), operates the nation's largest integrated direct health care delivery system. While Medicare, Medicaid, and the Children's Health Insurance Program (CHIP) are also publicly funded, most health care services under these programs are delivered by private providers in private facilities. In contrast, the VA health care system is a truly public health care system in that the federal government owns the medical facilities and employs the health care providers.[1]

The VA's health care system is organized into 21 geographically defined Veterans Integrated Service Networks (VISNs) (see **Appendix**). Although policies and guidelines are developed at VA headquarters, to be applied throughout the system, management authority for basic decision making and budgetary responsibilities are delegated to the VISNs. VHA's health care delivery network includes 153 hospitals (medical centers), 135 nursing homes, 803 community-based outpatient clinics (CBOCs), 6 independent outpatient clinics, and 271 Readjustment Counseling Centers (Vet Centers), which are supported by more than 242,000 employees.

In general, eligibility for VA health care is based on veteran status, service-connected disabilities or exposures, income, and other factors such as former prisoner of war (POW) status or receipt of the Purple Heart. As required by the Veterans Health Care Eligibility Reform Act of 1996 (P.L. 104-262), most veterans are required to enroll in the VA health care system to receive care. Once enrolled, veterans are assigned into one of the eight priority groups based on various criteria. For instance, veterans who are rated 50% or more service-connected disabled or who are unemployable due to service-connected disabilities are enrolled in Priority Group 1.[2] According to VA, there are approximately 23.1 million living veterans in the U.S. Of these, approximately 8.3 million (36%) were enrolled in the VA health care system, and over 5.0 million unique veteran patients received care from the VA in FY2009.[3]

Generally, veterans have a choice of where they receive their care. While some veterans rely more heavily on care through the VA health care system, the majority of veterans not enrolled in the VA health care system receive care through the private sector which is financed by Medicare, private health insurance, or the military health care system.[4] VHA is a direct health care provider, but it is not generally a third-party payer of care. For veterans who are eligible to receive care through the VA health care system, the decision on whether to receive care from the VA may depend on a variety of factors, such as out-of-pocket costs, distance, and waiting times for appointments, among other things.[5]

In general, VHA provides a majority of medical services to enrolled veterans within its health care system. However, in some instances, such as when a clinical service cannot be provided by a VA medical center, and the patient cannot be transferred to another VA medical facility; or when VA cannot recruit a needed clinician; or when a veteran is unable to access VA health care facilities due to geographic inaccessibility; or in emergencies when delays could lead to life threatening situations; VA is authorized to send the veteran outside of its health care system to seek care.[6]

VHA uses two major mechanisms to provide care outside its health care system. These include contracts to purchase care, or non-contracted medical care purchased on a fee for service basis from providers in the community. See the box below for a brief description of these methods.

Methods Used to Provide Care Outside the VA Health Care System

Contracts to Purchase Care: Generally, VA uses two approaches under this method. One is regular commercial contracts that follow Federal Acquisition Regulations, and are awarded on a competitive basis. The second is contracts or agreements with academic affiliates. VA's academic affiliates (schools of medicine, academic medical centers and their associated clinical practices) provide contracted clinical care. Generally, these are non-competitive sharing agreements, and details vary considerably from agreement to agreement. Most cover specialty services such as anesthesiology, cardiology, neurosurgery, ophthalmology, orthopedic surgery, or radiology. Sharing agreements can be based on full-time-equivalent (FTE) employment, or on specific procedures. Compared to fee basis care these contracts involve many patients, and are longer term contracts.

Fee Basis Care: Generally, fee basis care is used to provide outpatient care, and is authorized on a fee-for-service basis per episode of care. VA manages the authorization, claims processing and reimbursement for services acquired from non-VA health care providers. Fee basis care is sometimes referred to as "purchased care."

In 2006, Congress directed VHA to implement a contracting pilot program, which was later named Project Healthcare Effectiveness through Resource Optimization (Project HERO) to better manage the fee basis care program (discussed later in this chapter).

Policymakers and other stakeholders hold a variety of views regarding the appropriate role of the private sector in meeting the health care needs of eligible veterans. Some believe that the best course for veterans is to provide all needed care in facilities under the direct jurisdiction of the VA. On the other hand, some see the use of private sector providers as important in assuring veterans' access to a comprehensive slate of services (in particular, to specialty services that are needed infrequently), or in addressing geographic or other access barriers. In addition, those who believe that all needed care should be provided by VA providers in VA-owned facilities are concerned that private sector options for providing care to veterans will lead to a dilution of quality of care in the VA health care system, and could fail to leverage key strengths of the VHA network, such as its system of electronic medical records. However, some propose that over the long term, having private sector options could improve the quality of services within the VHA network through competition. Reaching the correct balance between providing care through VA's health care network and through non-VA providers is an issue for policymakers, as well as for the VHA and other stakeholders.

In addition to these broad concerns, Congress has been interested in specific aspects of VHA's use of private health care services. First, expenditures for contract and fee basis care services are increasing. In FY2008, VHA spent approximately $3.0 billion for contract and fee basis care. By FY2009, that amount had increased by 27% to approximately $3.8 billion.[7] These expenditures now comprise an estimated 9% of VHA's $41.9 billion total appropriations.[8]

Second, specific concerns have been raised about the fee basis care program. The program is complex, highly decentralized, and lacks a standardized implementation process across the VA health care system. Specifically, VA's Office of Inspector General (OIG) has reported that VHA has made a significant number of improper payments for fee basis care, and in some instances has not properly justified and authorized care.[9]

Congress established the Project HERO demonstration to determine if it could provide better management of non-VA provided care. At least two policy questions about Project HERO may be of interest to Congress:

1. Has Project HERO enhanced the existing fee basis care program? [10]
2. Are there findings from Project HERO that could be applied to standardize the fee basis care program throughout the VA health care system?

To provide some context to the discussion of these questions, this chapter first provides an overview of Project HERO. Second, it discusses the current fee basis care process, as well as the implementation of Project HERO. The report concludes with a discussion of observations on the implementation of Project HERO based on VHA and Humana Veterans Healthcare Services Inc. (HVHS) perspectives. This chapter is based on information received during visits to three of the four Project HERO demonstration sites as well as discussions with officials from HVHS.[11] Although the provision of dental care through Delta Dental Federal Services is part of Project HERO, this chapter does not discuss this aspect of the program.

PROJECT HEALTHCARE EFFECTIVENESS THROUGH RESOURCE OPTIMIZATION (PROJECT HERO)

As stated earlier, in 2006, Congress directed VHA to implement a contracting pilot program, to better manage the fee basis care program. The conference report (H.Rept. 109-305) to accompany the Military Quality of Life and Veterans Affairs Appropriations Act, 2006 (P.L. 109-114), directed the VA to implement a cost-effective purchased care management program and to develop at least three objectives-oriented demonstrations (pilot programs) to encourage collaboration with industry and academia. According to the conference report:

> The conferees support expeditious action by the Department to implement care management strategies that have proven valuable in the broader public and private sectors. It is essential that care purchased for enrollees from private sector providers be secured in a cost effective manner, in a way that complements the larger Veterans Health Administration system of care, and preserves an important agency interest, such as sustaining a partnership with university affiliates. In that interest, the VHA shall establish, through competitive award by the end of calendar year 2006, at least three managed care demonstration programs designed to satisfy a set of health system objectives related to arranging and managing care.[12]

The VA began developing plans based on this requirement. However, although the conference report language directed VA to implement a managed care demonstration, after meetings with various stakeholders VHA developed a set of objectives that led to a demonstration program to enhance the existing fee basis care program. Its goals were to[13]

- provide as much care for veterans within the VHA system as possible;
- when necessary, efficiently refer veterans to high-quality community-based care;
- improve exchange of information between VA and community providers;
- increase veteran patient satisfaction;
- foster high-quality care and patient safety;
- sustain partnership with university affiliates; and
- secure an accountable evaluation of demonstration results.

To implement this demonstration VHA selected four Veterans Integrated Service Networks (VISNs),[14] based on data that showed that these four networks had the highest expenditures for community-based care relative to the number of veterans enrolled for care. In addition, these areas included some of VHA's largest networks representing 25% of VHA's total enrollment.[15] A contract for medical services was awarded on October 1, 2007, to Humana Veterans Healthcare Services Inc. (HVHS).[16] Medical, surgical, mental health, diagnostic, and dialysis services became available through a network of providers recruited by HVHS. The demonstration program became operational on January 1, 2008.

OVERVIEW OF FEE BASIS CARE[17]

Services provided in non-VA health care facilities and by non-VA providers fall into two broad categories: contract care and fee basis care. Since Project HERO is a pilot to enhance fee basis care, this part of the report will first provide an overview of the current fee basis care process in the VHA. Under this system VA health care facilities are authorized to pay for health care services acquired from non-VA health care providers. VA manages the authorization, claims processing and reimbursement for services acquired from non-VA health care providers through the fee basis care program.[18]

The fee basis care program is used predominantly to provide outpatient care. Outpatient fee care involves two major phases: (1) pre-authorization of care and (2) claims processing. **Figure 1** provides a generalized depiction of the pre-authorization phase.

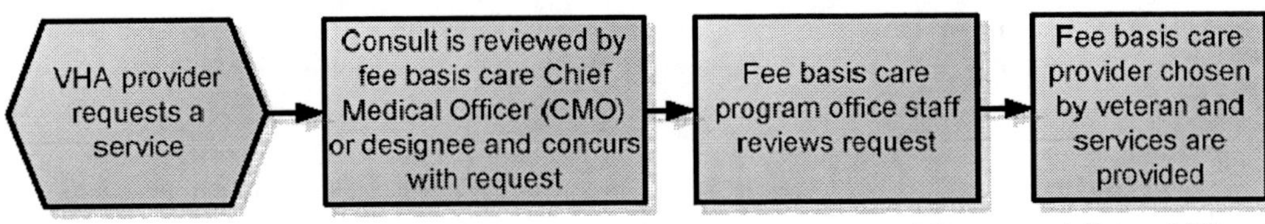

Source: Congressional Research Service graphic based on Department of Veterans Affairs, Office of Inspector General, *Audit of Veterans Health Administration's Non-VA Outpatient Fee Care Program*, Report No. 08-02901-185, Washington, DC, August 23, 2009, p. 20, and Project HERO briefing by Alvin S. Haynes Jr., M.D., Chief Medical Officer, Fee Basis Program, Bay Pines VA Health Care System, April 22, 2009.

Figure 1. Non-VA Outpatient Fee Basis Care, Pre-Authorization Phase.

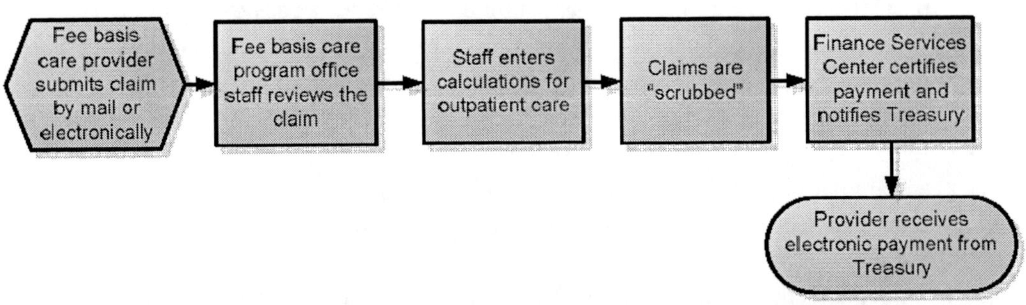

Source: Congressional Research Service graphic based on Department of Veterans Affairs, Office of Inspector General, Audit of Veterans Health Administration's Non-VA Outpatient Fee Care Program, Report No. 08-02901-185, Washington, DC, August 23, 2009, p. 20, and Project HERO briefing by Alvin S. Haynes Jr., M.D., Chief Medical Officer, Fee Basis Program, Bay Pines VA Health Care System, April 22, 2009.

Notes: Claims "scrubbing" broadly means a process whereby medical claims are validated against a set of established rules such as correct diagnostic codes (International Classification of Diseases, 9th Revision; ICD-9 codes) and procedure codes (such as Current Procedural Terminology (CPT) codes—a list of descriptive terms and identifying codes for reporting medical services and procedures).

Figure 2. Receipt and Processing of Fee Claims.

As seen in **Figure 1** a VA health care provider (generally a clinician) requests a specific health care service or procedure for the veteran and justifies use of non-VA care because of the lack of clinical capacity or capability to provide the service to the veteran. After the initial consult is received by the fee basis care program office at the local VA medical center (VAMC), the Chief Medical Officer (CMO) at the program office, or a designated official, reviews the request and authorizes the care if it is determined to be appropriate. Following this first stage of review, fee basis care program office staff reviews the authorization. They review it to see if the veteran is eligible for the program and whether an appropriate justification has been provided. Once the veteran is notified that the service is authorized, he or she selects a provider and receives services.

The next phase of the fee basis care program is the processing of fee claims. **Figure 2** provides a generalized depiction of receipt and payment of claims.

Once the veteran receives care from a non-VA provider, the provider sends a claim to the fee basis care program office at the VAMC that authorized the care. The fee basis care program office staff then reviews the claim to ensure that billed services match the services that were authorized. Following this review, staff determines the correct pricing methodology and payment rate based on the type and location of care provided. In the next step the claims are "scrubbed," or validated, to ensure that they are properly coded. After this step staff releases the claim to the Finance Services Center in Austin, Texas to certify fee disbursements to the Department of the Treasury, and the non-VA provider receives an electronic payment.

How Project HERO Works Compared to Fee Basis Care

Under Project HERO, veterans receive primary care at their local VA health care facility, as is the case under the regular fee basis care program. Similarly, if a VA health care provider determines that the specific medical expertise or technology is not readily available at the local facility then the provider requests that the service be obtained from a non-VA provider. The consult request is reviewed by the fee basis care CMO and, if the CMO concurs, the request proceeds to the fee basis care program office. At this point in the process, the fee basis care program office determines whether to send the referral to Project HERO (based on whether the services are provided within a reasonable distance under Project HERO), and if so sends an authorization for care to HVHS.[19]

Generally, authorizations are provided to HVHS for each episode of required care. In contrast to the regular fee basis care program in which the veteran selects his or her own provider, under Project HERO HVHS contacts the veteran by phone to schedule an appointment with an HVHS network provider. During this process appointment details are communicated back to the referring VA health care facility, and the veteran receives a letter with appointment details and instructions. According to HVHS officials, the veteran receives a reminder call prior to the appointment.

HVHS coordinates the transfer of any required pre-visit clinical information from the local VA medical facility to the HVHS network provider. After the veteran is seen by the HVHS network provider, and if additional services are needed, HVHS sends a request back to the referring VAMC for authorization. Under the contract, HVHS is required to return clinical information from the visit back to the referring VA medical facility—typically within 30 days of the appointment. In contrast to regular fee basis care, where clinical information is received directly from the non-VA provider to the referring medical facility, under Project HERO all clinical information is channeled through HVHS. When possible, the information is returned in an electronic format. Otherwise, the information is sent through fax or in hard copy format. Once the clinical information is received, the referring VA medical center reviews it for coordination of care and uploads it into the Computerized Patient Record System (CPRS).[20] Timely return of clinical information to the referring VA medical center is not a requirement under the regular fee-basis care program. Moreover, there is a simplification of claims payment under Project HERO compared to the regular fee basis care process (see **Figure 2**), whereby under Project HERO the network provider submits a claim to HVHS and is paid within about 30 days, and HVHS then submits electronic claims to VA for payment. A general depiction of this process is provided in **Figure 3** and **Figure 4**.

PROJECT HERO IMPLEMENTATION

This section provides a brief overview of implementation of the Project HERO demonstration in the four pilot VISNs. This section will discuss utilization of the program compared to regular fee basis care and VA provided care, quality of care under Project HERO, and reimbursement and cost of care under the demonstration program.

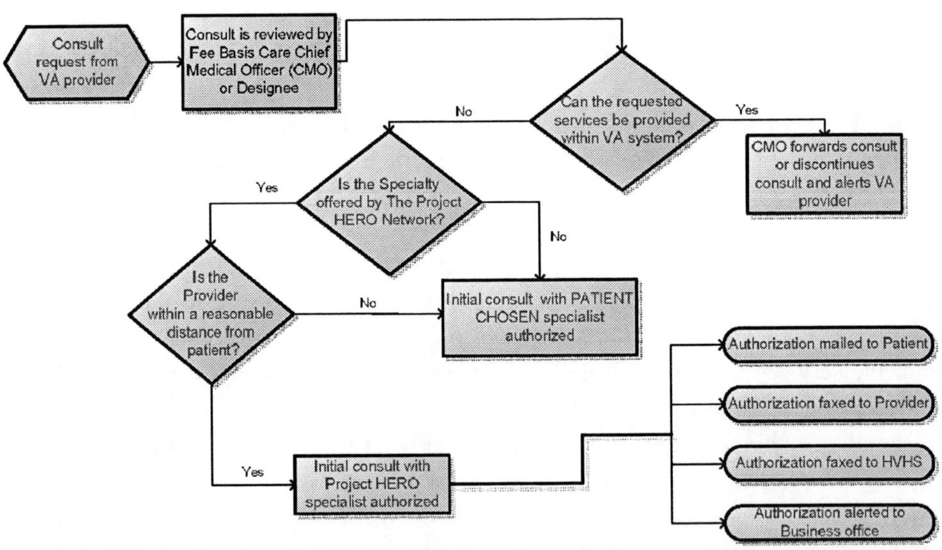

Source: : Congressional Research Service graphic based on Department of Veterans Affairs, Office of Inspector General, Audit of Veterans Health Administration's Non-VA Outpatient Fee Care Program, Report No. 08-02901-185, Washington, DC, August 23, 2009, p. 20, and Project HERO briefing by Alvin S. Haynes Jr., M.D., Chief Medical Officer, Fee Basis Program, Bay Pines VA Health Care System.

Notes: HVHS is Humana Veterans Health Care Services Inc. Also note that this a generalized depiction and the decision making process could vary from location to location.

Figure 3. Authorization Process For Non-VA Care Under Project HERO.

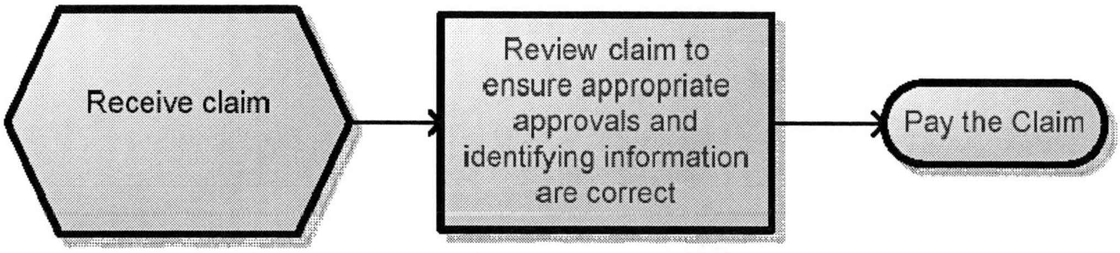

Source: Congressional Research Service graphic based on Project HERO briefing by Alvin S. Haynes Jr., M.D., Chief Medical Officer, Fee Basis Program, Bay Pines VA Health Care System, April 22, 2009.

Figure 4. Receipt and Processing of Fee Claims Under Project HERO.

Utilization

Project HERO is primarily an outpatient program. According to VHA data, between January 2008 and September 30, 2009, approximately 51,000 veteran patients received care through Project HERO within the four participating VISNs, compared to approximately 481,000 patients who received care through VHA's regular fee basis care program (**Figure 5**). During this same time period there were approximately 111,000 outpatient visits under Project HERO authorizations compared to approximately 1.8 million outpatient visits under regular fee basis care authorizations (**Figure 6**). As seen in the figures below, Project HERO represents a small percentage of all outpatient medical care provided by VHA.

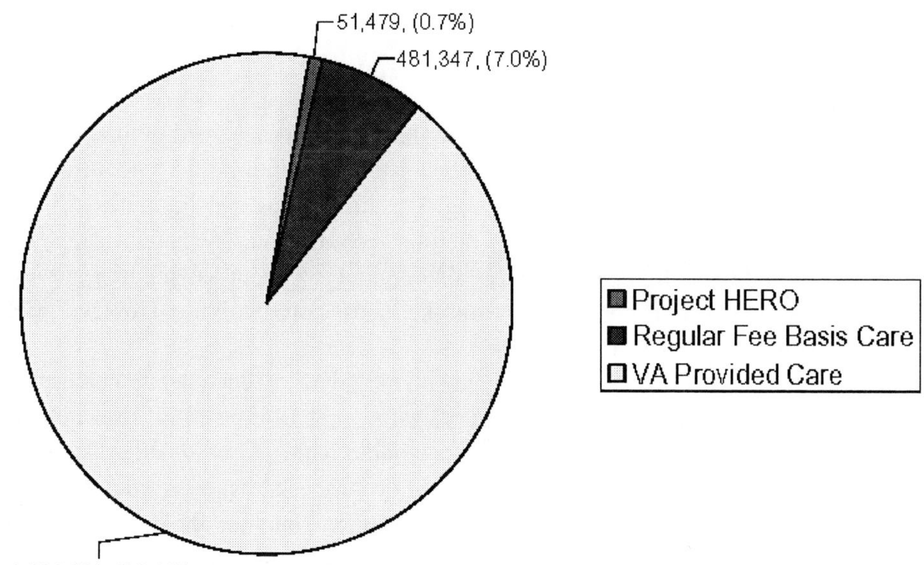

Source: Chart prepared by Congressional Research Service based on data from Department of Veterans Affairs, Veterans Health Administration, Chief Business Office.

Notes: Outpatient care provided from January 1, 2008 thru September 30, 2009.

Figure 5. Number and Percent Distribution of Unique Veteran Patients Receiving Outpatient Care (Total Patients in VISNs 8,16, 20, and 23).

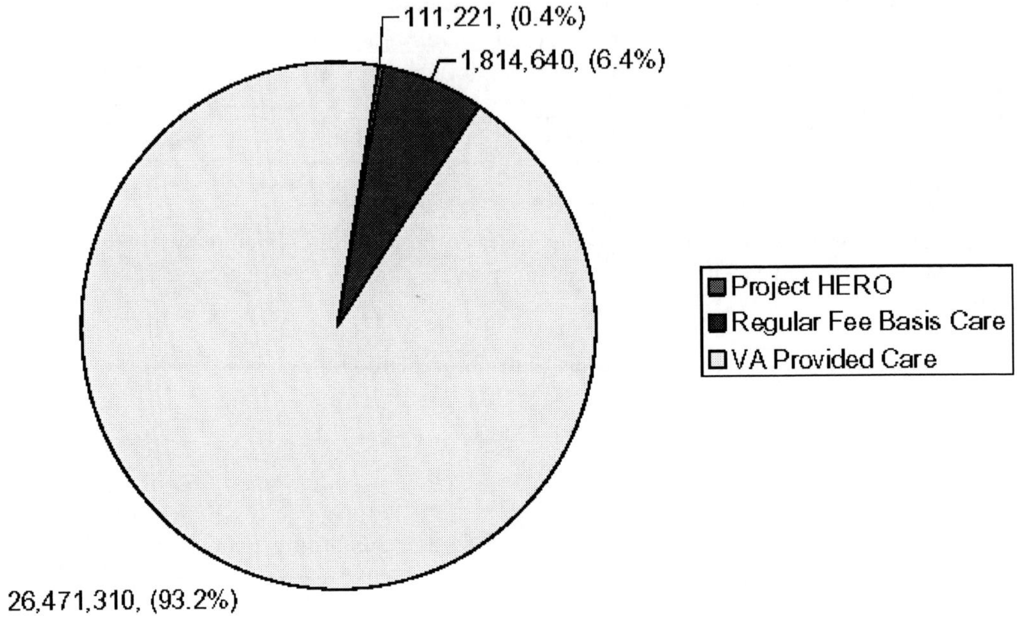

Source: : Chart prepared by Congressional Research Service based on data from Department of Veterans Affairs, Veterans Health Administration, Chief Business Office.
Notes: Outpatient visits from January 1, 2008 thru September 30, 2009.

Figure 6. Number and Percent Distribution of Outpatient Visits (Total Outpatient Visits in VISNs 8,16, 20, and 23).

Quality of Care

One objective for Project HERO is to ensure that veterans receive high quality care, even when that care is provided by non-VA providers in the community. The Project HERO demonstration includes measures of care along five dimensions: (1) timeliness of access to care, (2) return of clinical information, (3) facility accreditation, (4) patient safety, and (5) complaints.[21] In addition, the demonstration also conducts patient satisfaction surveys. The demonstration project is in its early stages, and the metrics are evolving. However, CRS was able to obtain some preliminary information.

Project HERO is used to provide quality health care when needed health care services are not available. "Not available" means that services are not offered at all, are not available within a reasonable amount of time, or are not available within a reasonable distance, within the VA health care system. Currently, VHA policy has established a goal of scheduling appointments within 30 days of the desired appointment but not more than four months beyond the desired appointment date. When a specific appointment date is not requested, VHA policy requires the scheduler to use the next available appointment. Furthermore, VHA policy also requires that all appointment requests, including consult referrals to a specialist, must be acted on by the medical facility within seven days.[22] The contract requires that HVHS report the following metrics as part of the standard evaluation of access to care: number of times care is provided within 30 days, number of appointments scheduled within 5 days, and number of patients seen within 20 minutes of appointment time. HVHS reports that in August 2009, 93.9 % of appointments were scheduled within five days of receipt of authorization, and that the average time it took to schedule an appointment was 2.1 business days once an authorization was received. HVHS also claims that in the same month 88.2% of the referred patients were seen by a HVHS provider within 30 days.[23]

Under Project HERO, VHA did not establish drive time or distance requirements in the contract with HVHS. However, due to the need for such a standard, a business process has been mutually agreed upon by VHA and HVHS. HVHS notifies the referring VA medical center if the care provider is more than 50 miles from the veteran's home address. The referring VA medical center can determine if it is a reasonable distance based on where the veteran lives. If the VA medical center staff believes they can obtain care closer to the veteran, they can cancel the HVHS authorization and issue a regular fee basis care authorization.

With respect to the return of clinical information, under the Project HERO demonstration HVHS is required to provide clinical data generated as result of a routine referral for authorized care to the referring medical facility within 30 days of the appointment date, although this is not a requirement under the regular fee basis care program. Early reports from the Project HERO Program Management Office indicated that HVHS did not meet the 100% standard, and showed a downward trend in this measure, meaning that the percentage of records returned within 30 days was declining.[24] In September 2009, HVHS claimed that it was working on process improvements and on educating noncompliant providers. HVHS reported in August that average business days to return clinical information is 14.3 days.[25]

Accreditation of facilities and credentialing of providers are seen as proxy measures to evaluate quality of clinical care provided. Generally, under the regular fee basis care program, once a veteran is authorized to receive care outside the VA health care system, the veteran is free to choose a provider within the community. Therefore, although the provider may be licensed to practice medicine within the state, he or she is not necessarily credentialed in a manner similar to the credentialing process that VHA uses to credential its own health care providers.[26] However, under Project HERO requirements, HVHS has stated that it recruits credentialed providers using the same guidelines that VHA uses for its providers. Credentialing includes verification of appropriate education, certificates, licensing, criminal record, registrations and insurance. According to HVHS it only sends veterans to providers who meet VA credentialing requirements.[27] In addition, the Project HERO HVHS network of providers is required to practice at Joint Commission accredited facilities. Currently all facilities providing inpatient care within the contractor network are accredited by one of the following organizations: The Joint Commission, the Commission on Accreditation of Rehabilitation Facilities (CARF), The Intersocietal Commission for the Accreditation of Vascular Laboratories (ICVAL), or the American Osteopathic Association (AOA). According to the VA, the Project HERO Program Management Office audits HVHS for provider credentialing and facility accreditation, and to date, the VA has stated that the audit results have shown that HVHS providers are compliant with credentialing requirements.

According to the VHA National Patient Improvement Handbook, patient safety is ensuring freedom from accidental or inadvertent injury during health care processes.[28] Under Project HERO patient safety incidents must be reported within one business day to the referring VA medical facility, and these violations are required to be investigated and resolved by VHA and HVHS. In its July 2009 monthly report, the Project HERO Program Management Office did not report any patient safety violations.

With respect to complaints, a majority of complaints in the July 2009 report were related to the authorization process. For example: "one veteran was sent to a provider who could not perform the procedure needed," "another veteran had an appointment rescheduled and his medical records were not requested," and "another veteran went to an appointment and was told that the appointment was not scheduled for him."[29]

As part of Project HERO, HVHS conducts surveys of patients to measure patient satisfaction, and these are reported to the Project HERO Program Management Office. In its July 2009 report (representing averaged data from October 2008-March 2009), the Project HERO Program Management Office indicated that over 75% of patients were very or completely satisfied with their visit and 80% rated the overall quality of the visit as very good or excellent. However, only 52% were satisfied with their appointment wait times.[30]

Costs and Reimbursements

Project HERO prices for medical care are a negotiated percentage of U.S. Department of Health and Human Services (HHS), Centers for Medicare and Medicaid Services (CMS) rates based on the local market rates where the services are provided. In contrast, under the regular fee basis care, with the exception of physician services, dialysis and laboratory testing, VHA does not have authority to pay at CMS rates. VHA pays for regular fee basis outpatient care based on the lesser of the amount billed by the provider or the amount calculated using a formula developed by CMS's participating physician fee schedule for the period in which the service is provided. If there is no calculated amount under the CMS's participating physician fee schedule, reimbursements are based on the lesser of the actual amount billed or the amount calculated using the VA's 75th percentile methodology or the usual and customary rate.[31] Under Project HERO, VHA pays HVHS a value added fee that ranges from $30.75 to $48.09 per claim, and these amounts vary by VISN and type of service (see **Table 1**).

The value added fee supports provision of such services as: coordinating appointments for veterans; returning clinical information (for example medical records) to VHA; processing provider invoices for reimbursement to providers; and monitoring and reporting access to care, appointment timeliness and patient safety. As seen in **Table 2**, in FY2008 VHA paid approximately $69,000, and for FY2009 it paid HVHS approximately $3.3 million in value added fees.

Table 1. Value Added Fee Amounts, FY2009

	VISN 8	VISN 16	VISN 20	VISN 23
Medical or Surgical Care Services	$30.75	$30.75	$39.50	$39.24
Mental Health Care Services	$36.89	$36.89	$45.74	$48.09
Diagnostic Services	$30.75	$30.75	$39.50	$39.24
Dialysis	$30.75	$30.75	$39.50	$39.24

Source: Humana Veterans Healthcare Services.

Table 2. Project HERO Payments Including Value Added Fees

	Project HERO Payments for Health Care, excluding Value-Added Fees[a]	Project HERO Value Added Fees[b]	Total Project HERO Payments	Value Added Fees as a % of Project HERO Payments	VISN Budgets[c]	Total Project HERO payments as % of VISN Budgets
FY2008	$5,223,422	$69,089	$5,292,511	1.30%	$8,973,617,617	0.06%
FY2009	$38,669,257	$3,305,067	$41,974,324	7.87%	$9,685,045,154	0.43%

Source: Department of Veterans Affairs, Veterans Health Administration, Chief Business Office.

Notes: a. Project HERO Payments are VHA payments to Humana Veterans Health Care Services Inc. excluding any value added fees (VISNs 8, 16, 20, and 23), and do not include dental care payments to Delta Dental. Payments for FY2008 are from January 2008 through September 2008, and payments for FY2009 are from October 1, 2008 through September 30, 2009.

b. Value added fees are payments made by VHA to Humana Veterans Health Care Services Inc (HVHS) for services such as coordinating appointments for veterans; returning clinical information to VHA on a timely basis; processing provider invoices for quick reimbursement to providers; and monitoring and reporting access to care, appointment, timeliness and patient safety. Data are based on HVHS reporting of value added fees.

c. FY2008 VISN budgets (total VISN budgets for 8, 16, 20, and 23) are obligations as of September 30, 2008 and FY2009 VISN budgets are as of July 31, 2009.

DISCUSSION

Stakeholders have voiced various concerns about care provided outside the VA health care system, and these concerns have been voiced regarding both contract care and fee basis care. Some Veterans Service Organizations (VSO) are concerned that a mixture of government providers and private providers could grow over time and place at risk the VA health care system as a whole.[32] Unions are concerned that care provided by non-VA providers would eventually lead to "outsourcing of functions that have traditionally been performed in-house."[33]

Congress has expressed concern with the growth of non-VA provided care, and whether VHA is prudently using taxpayer dollars to purchase care for veterans. Congress has also expressed concern about whether VHA can ensure timely access to quality care when that care is provided by outside providers.[34] The Project HERO demonstration is characterized by the VA as an effort to address these concerns and in the early stage of its implementation is perceived to have achieved mixed results. The next part of this chapter addresses the two questions posed at the beginning of this chapter.

Has Project HERO Enhanced the Fee Basis Care Program?

During visits to three of the four demonstration sites CRS heard mixed reviews about the pilot program. Some categorized it as a "tool in a toolbox" meaning that Project HERO was one of many options a VA medical facility could use to provide care outside the VA health care system (other options include care through medical school affiliates or through existing contracts with local providers, among others). Some officials categorized Project HERO as a "concierge service" where HVHS guides the veterans in scheduling appointments and ensuring that clinical information is provided to a network provider and then transferred back to the VA, as well as maintaining a credentialed network of providers, and claims payment to providers.

The current Project HERO demonstration could be categorized as an enhancement of the regular fee basis care program. The demonstration pilot provides a single point of contact for those veterans who are authorized to receive care outside the VA health care system. Under the demonstration HVHS works with the veterans and the HVHS network provider in scheduling the appointment. It also allows the veteran to seek care from a credentialed provider, as well as facilitates the transfer of medical information, thereby assisting with care coordination. Furthermore, under Project HERO, VA does not have the responsibility for paying for care provided outside the system directly to non-VA providers. However, VA pays for these services through value added fees to HVHS.

Are There Lessons to Be Learned from the Pilot Program?

(1) Establishing a robust network of providers takes time, even when dealing with an established health care services provider.
Most VISNs stated that early on in the pilot HVHS had fair to moderate success building its network of providers within the VISN, and that the short implementation period between the time the contract was awarded in October 2007 to when it became operational in January 2008, was inadequate to establish a robust network of providers. This was especially true in VISNs that had rural or highly rural areas. According to some VISN officials, in some instances this lack of a network of providers has resulted in ongoing challenges in providing timely access to medical care. HVHS has asserted that based on feedback received from the Project HERO Program Management Office, it has worked with VA to resolve most of these issues. For example, HVHS has adapted to the changing clinical needs of each VISN and has attempted to recruit a provider network to meet those clinical needs.

(2) Establishing services and pricing, and keeping them up-to-date, is a challenge.
Some VISNs stated that clinical care services included in the contract were based on prior needs and did not meet the current needs of the network. Some VISNs also raised the issue that some contract pricing is higher than what VA would have paid under the regular fee basis care, and that some services are cost-prohibitive when the value-added fees are applied. However, the Project HERO Program Management Office has noted that 89% of Project HERO prices are at or below CMS rates, and

that amounts paid to providers are less than 7% of the regular fee basis care program.[35]

(3) Education is key to a successful functioning network.
Almost all VISNs stated that there has been organizational resistance to change. According to VISN staff, the primary implementation challenge has been providing training to staff at all levels of the organization, especially educating providers and fee basis care office staff. This has been true even for providers recruited by HVHS, especially when they are required to send clinical information back to the VA.

(4) The project has yielded information that could be applied to the existing regular fee basis care program.
First, without the electronic sharing of medical records between the VA health care system and non-VA providers, there are delays in the transfer of clinical information. In some instances this delay may result in a VA provider not being alerted to the need for immediate follow-up care required based on a diagnosis or laboratory result. Second, VHA's regular fee basis care program could adopt certain quality metrics that are currently used under Project HERO, such as how far the veteran travels to receive his or her care as well as how long the veteran waits once he or she arrives for an appointment. Lastly, VA could develop a provider network within each VISN that the veteran could be referred to so that the veteran receives care from provider who has been credentialed similarly to a VA provider. However, prior to implementing this pilot demonstration throughout the VA health care system, it may be useful to conduct an independent evaluation to conclusively measure if Project HERO has been a worthwhile effort.

APPENDIX. VETERANS INTEGRATED SERVICES NETWORKS (VISNS)

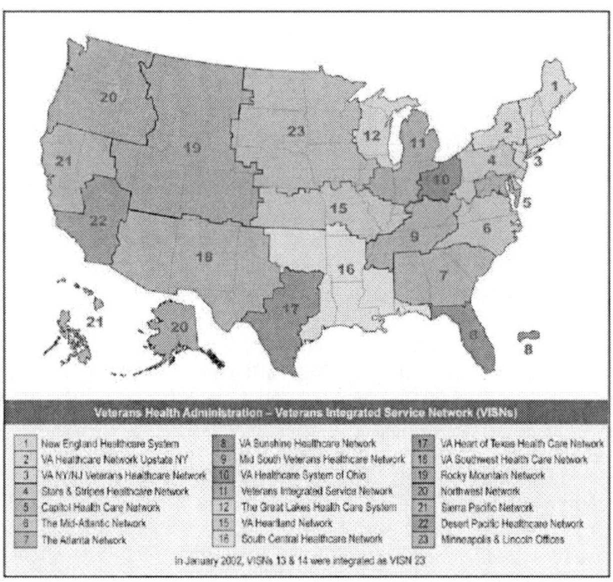

Source: Department of Veterans Affairs, adapted by Congressional Research Service.

End Notes

[1] U.S. Congress, House, *Economic Report of the President,* 110th Cong., 2nd sess., February 2008, H. Doc. 110-83 (Washington: GPO, 2008), p. 106.

[2] For a complete discussion of eligibility for VA health care, priority groups, and enrollment, see CRS Report R40737, *Veterans Medical Care: FY2010 Appropriations*, by Sidath Viranga Panangala.

[3] Department of Veterans Affairs, *FY2009 Performance and Accountability Report*, Washington, DC, November 16, 2009, pp. I-16- I17.

[4] Congressional Budget Office, *Quality Initiatives Undertaken by the Veterans Health Administration*, August 2009, p. 5. Veterans who are military retirees have access to TRICARE, the Department of Defense health care plan. For more information, see CRS Report RL33537, *Military Medical Care: Questions and Answers*, by Don J. Jansen, and CRS Report RS22402, *Increases in Tricare Costs: Background and Options for Congress*, by Don J. Jansen.

[5] Congressional Budget Office, *Quality Initiatives Undertaken by the Veterans Health Administration*, August 2009, p.7.

[6] 38 U.S.C. §1703 authorizes non-VA inpatient and outpatient medical services on a preauthorized basis by contract or individual authorization; 38 U.S.C. §1725 authorizes reimbursement for emergency treatment of nonservice-connected conditions in a non-VA facility without prior authorization; 38 U.S.C. §1728 authorizes reimbursement for emergency treatment of service-connected or related conditions in a non-VA facility without prior authorization.

[7] U.S. Congress, Senate Committee on Veterans' Affairs, *A Hearing on VA's Contracts for Health Services*, 111th Cong., 1st sess., September 30, 2009. Answer provided by Gary Baker, Chief Business Officer,Veterans Health Administration, U.S. Department of Veterans Affairs, to a question posed by Senator Daniel Akaka.

[8] CRS Report R40737, *Veterans Medical Care: FY2010 Appropriations*, by Sidath Viranga Panangala.

[9] Department of Veterans Affairs, Office of Inspector General, *Audit of Veterans Health Administration's Non-VA Outpatient Fee Care Program*, Report No. 08-02901-185, Washington, DC, August 23, 2009, pp. 4-10.

[10] S.Rept. 111-40 to accompany the Military Construction and Veterans Affairs and Related Agencies Appropriations Act, 2010 (S. 1407) expressed concern about the oversight and scope of Project HERO. See U.S. Congress, Senate Committee on Appropriations, *Military Construction and Veterans Affairs and Related Agencies Appropriation Bill, 2010*, report to accompany S. 1407, 111th Cong., 1st sess., July 7, 2009, p. 53.

[11] To better understand Project HERO implementation, on April 22, 2009, August 7, 2009, and August 26, 2009, Congressional Research Service (CRS) staff visited VISNs 8, 16, and 20 respectively. CRS staff did not visit VISN 23. During these meetings, CRS staff received briefings from VHA program staff at the respective VISNs, and held discussions on how the project has been implemented within each VISN. Lastly, on September 17, 2009, CRS staff spoke with officials of Humana Veterans Health Care Services Inc. (HVHS).

[12] U.S. Congress, Conference Committee, *Making Appropriations for Military Quality of Life Functions, of the Department Of Defense, Military Construction, the Department Of Veterans Affairs, and Related Agencies for The Fiscal Year Ending September 30, 2006, and for Other Purposes*, Report to accompany H.R. 2528, 109th Cong., 1st sess., November 18, 2005, H.Rept. 109-305, pp. 43-44.

[13] Based on briefings provided to CRS Staff by VISN 16 and VISN 20 program staff on August 7, 2009, and August 26, 2009 respectively. For a list of initial objectives see U.S. Congress, House Committee on Veterans' Affairs, *Project Healthcare Effectiveness Through Resource Optimization*, 109th Cong., 2nd sess., March 29, 2006 (Washington: GPO, 2007), p. 66.

[14] The VA's health care system is organized into 21 geographically defined Veterans Integrated Service Networks (VISNs). Although policies and guidelines are developed at VA headquarters to be applied throughout the VA health care system, management authority for basic decision making and budgetary responsibilities is delegated to the VISNs (see Kenneth Kizer, John Demakis, and John Feussner, "Reinventing VA Health Care: Systematizing Quality Improvement and Quality Innovation." *Medical Care*. vol. 38, no. 6 (June 2000), Suppl 1:I7-16.

[15] U.S. Congress, House Committee on Veterans' Affairs, *Project Healthcare Effectiveness Through Resource Optimization*, 109th Cong., 2nd sess., March 29, 2006 (Washington: GPO, 2007), p. 16.

[16] The VA contract with HVHS is an indefinite delivery, indefinite quantity (IDIQ) one-year contract with four option years. In general, an IDIQ contract is a type of indefinite delivery contract that provides for an indefinite quantity of supplies or services within stated limits, during a fixed period. The government places orders for individual requirements.Quantity limits may be stated as number of units or as dollar values. Federal Acquisition Regulation (FAR) 16.504.

[17] Major portions of this section were drawn from Department of Veterans Affairs, Office of Inspector General, *Audit of Veterans Health Administration's Non-VA Outpatient Fee Care Program*, Report No. 08-02901-185, Washington, DC, August 23, 2009, pp. 20-21.

[18] The fee basis care program is sometimes referred to as the purchased care program.

[19] It should be noted that each of the pilot VISNs has inter-and intra-VISN referral policies. For example, if a specific VA medical facility cannot provide the required services, the next step would be to see if another facility within the VISN, and within reasonable distance to the veteran, could provide that specific service or if an academic affiliate or Department of Defense (DOD) sharing agreement could be used to provide that service. If these options are not available then the referring VA medical facility could authorize the use of Project HERO or non-Project HERO fee basis care.

[20] The CPRS is a single integrated system for VA health care providers, and a package within the Veterans Health Information Systems and Technology Architecture (VistA). All aspects of a patient's medical record are integrated, including active problems, allergies, current medications, laboratory results, vital signs, hospitalizations and outpatient clinic history, alerts of abnormal results, among other things. It is used in about 1,300 VHA facilities around the country. CPRS also incorporates data from scheduling, laboratory, radiology, consults and clinic notes into a single integrated patient record.

[21] Department of Veterans Affairs, Veterans Health Administration, Chief Business Office, *Project HERO Demonstration Evaluation Monthly Report*, July 2009.

[22] U.S. Congress, House Committee on Veterans' Affairs, Subcommittee on Health and Subcommittee on Oversight and Investigations, *Outpatient Waiting Times*, 110th Cong., 1st sess., December 12, 2007. p.35.

[23] Humana Veterans Health Care Services briefing, September 17, 2009.

[24] Department of Veterans Affairs, Veterans Health Administration, Chief Business Office, *Project HERO Demonstration Evaluation Monthly Report*, July 2009.

[25] Humana Veterans Health Care Services briefing, September 17, 2009.

[26] VHA policy requires that all VHA health care professionals who are permitted by law and the facility to provide patient care services independently must be credentialed and privileged. Credentialing is done to ensure that a provider has the required education, training, experience, physical and mental health, and skill to fulfill the requirements of the position and to support the requested clinical privileges (see VHA HANDBOOK 1100.19, November 14, 2008).

[27] Humana Veterans Health Care Services briefing September 17, 2009.

[28] Department of Veterans Affairs, Veterans Health Administration, VHA HANDBOOK 1050.01, May 23, 2008.

[29] Department of Veterans Affairs, Veterans Health Administration, Chief Business Office, *Project HERO Demonstration Evaluation Monthly Report*, July 2009.

[30] Ibid, pp.9-11.

[31] 38 C.F.R. § 17.56. Reimbursement under the 75th percentile methodology is determined for each VA medical facility by ranking all treatment occurrences of a medical procedure (with a minimum of eight) under the corresponding Current Procedural Terminology (CPT®) codes during the previous fiscal year with charges ranked from the highest to the lowest rate billed and the charge falling at the 75th percentile as the maximum amount to be paid. If there are fewer than eight treatment occurrences for a procedure during the previous fiscal year then VA pays based on the provider's usual or customary charges.

[32] U.S. Congress, House Committee on Veterans' Affairs, *Project Healthcare Effectiveness Through Resource Optimization*, 109th Cong., 2nd sess., March 29, 2006 (Washington: GPO, 2007), p.76.

[33] U.S. Congress, Senate Committee on Veterans' Affairs, *A Hearing on VA's Contracts for Health Services*, 111th Cong., 1st sess., September 30, 2009. Testimony by Mary A. Curtis, Psychiatric Clinical Nurse Specialist and Clinical Application Coordinator Boise VA Medical Center Boise, Idaho, on Behalf of American Federation of Government Employees, AFL-CIO.

[34] U.S. Congress, Senate Committee on Veterans' Affairs, *A Hearing on VA's Contracts for Health Services*, 111th Cong., 1st sess., September 30, 2009.

[35] Communication received from Department of Veterans Affairs, Veterans Health Administration, Chief Business Office, September 29, 2009.

In: Veterans Benefits
Editors: George B. Meyers and Alice M. Glaskin

ISBN: 978-1-61209-581-3

Chapter 6

VETERANS AFFAIRS: HEALTH CARE AND BENEFITS FOR VETERANS EXPOSED TO AGENT ORANGE

Sidath Viranga Panangala and Douglas Reid Weimer

SUMMARY

Since the 1970s, Vietnam-era veterans have attributed certain medical illnesses, disabilities, and birth defects to exposure to Agent Orange and other herbicides sprayed by the U.S. Air Force to destroy enemy crops and remove forest cover. During the last 30 years, Agent Orange legislation has established and updated the health and disability benefits of Vietnam veterans exposed to herbicides.

Several laws were enacted by Congress to provide health care services to Vietnam veterans. The Veterans' Health Care, Training and Small Business Loan Act (P.L. 97-72) elevated Vietnam veterans' priority status for health care at Department of Veterans Affairs facilities by recognizing a veteran's own report of exposure as sufficient proof to receive medical care unless there was evidence to the contrary. The Veterans' Health Care Eligibility Reform Act of 1996 (P.L. 104-262) completely restructured the VA medical care eligibility requirements for all veterans. Under P.L. 104-262, a veteran does not have to demonstrate a link between a certain health condition and exposure to Agent Orange; instead, medical care is provided unless the VA has determined that the condition did not result from exposure to Agent Orange.

Likewise, Congress passed several measures to address disability compensation issues of Vietnam veterans. The Veterans' Dioxin and Radiation Exposure Compensation Standards Act of 1984 (P.L. 98-542) required the VA to develop regulations for disability compensation to Vietnam veterans exposed to Agent Orange. In 1991, the Agent Orange Act (P.L. 102-4) established for the first time a process for establishing presumption of service connection for diseases associated with herbicide exposure. P.L. 102-4 authorized the VA to contract with the Institute of Medicine (IOM) to conduct scientific reviews of the evidence linking certain medical conditions to herbicide exposure. Under this law, the VA is required to review the reports of the IOM and issue regulations, establishing a presumption of service connection for any disease for which there is scientific evidence of a positive association with herbicide exposure. Based on these IOM reports, currently 14 health conditions are presumptively service-connected, including B-cell leukemias, Parkinson's disease, and ischemic heart disease.

Navy veterans of the Vietnam Era (those who served in Vietnam between January 9, 1962, and May 7, 1975), who served offshore and were never physically present on Vietnamese soil, have been contesting the presumption of service connection for Agent Orange disability benefits. In 2006, the U.S. Court of Appeals for Veterans Claims (CAVC) ruled in *Haas v. Nicholson* that navy veterans who served offshore during the Vietnam Era were entitled to a presumption of exposure to Agent Orange. On May 8, 2008, the U.S. Court of Appeals for the Federal Circuit ("the court") issued a decision reversing the CAVC's decision. On June 23, 2008, the attorneys for Haas filed a petition with the court for a panel rehearing or a rehearing en banc (that is, the whole panel of judges of the court). On October 9, 2008, the court denied the petition. Following this action, Haas petitioned the U.S. Supreme Court for certiorari (asking the Supreme Court to review the decision of a lower court). On January 21, 2009, the Supreme Court denied the petition for writ of certiorari. A subsequent related proceeding, *Haas v. Shinseki*, on remand from the court, involved the same plaintiff and the same factual situation. On March 10, 2009, the court examined the BVA's decision, vacated that decision, and remanded the claim for further proceedings with the BVA. The Agent Orange Equity Act of 2009 (H.R. 2254), if enacted, would clarify service in Vietnam to include inland waterways, the waters offshore, and airspace above Vietnam. Under H.R. 2254, those who have been awarded the Vietnam Service Medal or the Vietnam Campaign Medal would also be eligible for disability compensation based on presumptive disease conditions relating to exposure to Agent Orange.

BACKGROUND

Between 1962 and 1971, the U.S. Air Force sprayed approximately 107 million pounds of herbicides in South Vietnam for the purpose of defoliation and crop destruction. The herbicides sprayed during the Vietnam era contained mixtures of 2,4-dichlorophenoxyacetic acid (2,4-D), 2,4,5-trichlorophenoxyacetic acid (2,4,5-T), picloram, and cacodylic acid. The most extensively used defoliant compound, a 50:50 combination of 2,4-D and 2,4,5-T, came to be known as "Agent Orange" because of the orange-colored band placed on each chemical storage container. One of the chemicals used in Agent Orange, 2,4,5-T, contained small amounts of dioxin. Other herbicides employed in Vietnam such as "Agent Purple" and "Agent Green" also were contaminated with dioxin. Collectively, these compounds were referred to as the "rainbow defoliants." The late 1960s saw a decline in the use of these herbicides when dioxin, already well known to be highly toxic in animals, was implicated in birth defects seen in mice. By 1969, spraying was restricted to remote areas, and by 1971, the Air Force ceased all spraying of Agent Orange.

Since the late 1970s, Vietnam-era veterans have voiced concerns about how exposure to Agent Orange may have affected their health and caused certain disabilities, including birth defects in their children. Initially, the Department of Defense (DOD) maintained that only a limited number of U.S. military personnel, such as those operating aircraft or troops engaged in herbicide spraying, could be positively linked to Agent Orange exposure. However, in 1979, the General Accounting Office, now the Government Accountability Office (GAO), reported that ground troops had also been exposed to Agent Orange, and DOD was forced to reconsider its prior statements.[1] In response to these concerns, Congress passed legislation to research the long-term health effects on Vietnam veterans and to provide benefits and services to those who may have been exposed to Agent Orange.[2]

This chapter provides an overview of health care services and disability compensation benefits available to Vietnam veterans, Children of Vietnam Era veterans, and non-Vietnam veterans exposed to herbicides. This is followed by a discussion of litigation pertaining to Navy veterans of the Vietnam Era who served offshore and were never physically present on Vietnamese soil. The report concludes with a discussion of epidemiologic research conducted to study the health effects of Agent Orange and dioxin exposure on Vietnam veterans.

HEALTH CARE

Prior to the 1981 Veterans' Health Care, Training and Small Business Loan Act (P.L. 97-72), veterans who complained of Agent Orange-related illnesses were generally at the lowest priority for treatment at Department of Veterans Affairs (VA) medical facilities because these conditions were not considered "service-connected."[3] P.L. 97-72 elevated Vietnam veterans' priority status for health care at VA facilities by recognizing a veteran's own report of exposure as sufficient proof to receive medical care unless there was evidence to the contrary. The Veterans' Health Care Eligibility Reform Act of 1996 (P.L. 104-262) completely restructured the VA medical care eligibility requirements for all veterans. Under P.L. 104-262, a veteran does not have to demonstrate a link between a certain health condition and exposure to Agent Orange; instead, medical care is provided unless the VA has determined that the condition did not result from exposure to Agent Orange or the condition has been identified by the Institute of Medicine (IOM) as having "limited/suggestive" evidence of *no* association between the occurrence of the disease and exposure to a herbicide.[4] The research by the IOM (part of the National Academies) and its significance is addressed later in this chapter.[5]

PRESUMPTION OF SERVICE CONNECTION

Prior to discussing disability compensation for exposure to Agent Orange, it is essential to provide a brief overview of presumptive service connection. In general, a veteran is entitled to compensation for disabilities incurred during active military service. There are several ways to establish that a disability is service-connected. The application of statutory presumptions is only one way to invoke compensation for a service-connected disability.[6] In the context of VA claims adjudication, a presumption could be seen as a procedure to relieve veterans of the burden to prove that a disability or illness was caused by a specific exposure that occurred during service in the Armed Forces. In other words, the onus is placed on the VA rather than the veteran. Most presumptions are applied to chronic disease or illnesses that manifest after a period of time following service.[7]

DISABILITY COMPENSATION

The Veterans' Dioxin and Radiation Exposure Compensation Standards Act of 1984 (P.L. 98-542) required the VA to develop regulations for disability compensation to Vietnam veterans who may have been exposed to Agent Orange. Veterans seeking compensation for a condition they thought to be related to herbicide exposure had to provide proof of a service connection that established the link between herbicide exposure and disease onset. P.L. 98-542 authorized disability compensation payments to Vietnam veterans for the skin condition chloracne, which is associated with herbicide exposure. In 1991, the Agent Orange Act (P.L. 102-4) established for the first time a process for establishing presumption of service connection for diseases associated with herbicide exposure. P.L. 102-4 authorized the VA to contract with the IOM to review and summarize the scientific evidence concerning the association between exposure to herbicides used in support of military operations in Vietnam during the Vietnam Era and each disease suspected to be associated with such exposure. P.L. 102-4 mandated that IOM determine, to the extent possible: (1) whether there is a statistical association between the suspect diseases and herbicide exposure, taking into account the strength of the scientific evidence and the appropriateness of the methods used to detect the association; (2) the increased risk of disease among individuals exposed to herbicides during service in Vietnam during the Vietnam Era; and (3) whether there is a plausible biological mechanism or other evidence of a causal relationship between herbicide exposure and the health outcome.[8] The VA is then required to review the reports of the IOM and issue regulations, establishing a presumption of service connection for any disease for which there is scientific evidence of a positive association with herbicide exposure. Once the VA has established presumption of service connection for a certain disease or medical condition, a Vietnam veteran with that disease is eligible for disability compensation. The amount of compensation is based on the degree of disability and, again, veterans are compensated only for approved conditions that have demonstrated sufficient evidence of an association with herbicide exposure.[9] The next three sections provide information on diseases that are currently presumptively service-connected for Agent Orange, diseases that have not been recognized as presumptively service-connected, and benefits available for children of Vietnam-era veterans.

Diseases Associated with Exposure to Certain Herbicide Agents

Currently, the conditions that are presumptively recognized for service connection for Vietnam veterans are chloracne (must occur within one year of exposure to Agent Orange); non-Hodgkin's lymphoma; soft tissue sarcoma (other than osteosarcoma, chondrosarcoma, Kaposi's sarcoma, or mesothelioma); Hodgkin's disease; porphyria cutanea tarda (must occur within one year of exposure); multiple myeloma; respiratory cancers, including cancers of the lung, larynx, trachea, and bronchus; prostate cancer; acute and subacute transient peripheral neuropathy (must appear within one year of exposure and resolve within two years of date of onset); type II diabetes; chronic lymphocytic leukemia (CLL);[10] amyotrophic lateral sclerosis (ALS);[11] and AL amyloidosis.[12]

Recent Additions to the List of Presumptive Disease Conditions

On October 13, 2009, the VA issued a press release stating that it would establish a presumptive service connection for three specific illnesses based on the IOM report *Veterans and Agent Orange: Update 2008.*[13] The illnesses affected by the VA decision are B-cell leukemias, such as hairy cell leukemia; Parkinson's disease; and ischemic heart disease.[14] On March 25, 2010, the VA issued proposed regulations[15] establishing these presumptions, and final regulations were issued on August 31, 2010.[16]

The Congressional Review Act and the New Presumptive Disease Conditions[17]

Although final rules were issued on August 31, section 902 of the Supplemental Appropriations Act, 2010 (P.L. 111-212) contained a provision limiting the VA from spending any funds provided in P.L. 111-212, on disability compensation for veterans exposed to Agent Orange and diagnosed with hairy cell leukemia and other chronic B cell leukemias, Parkinson's disease, and ischemic heart disease, until the expiration of the congressional review period under the Congressional Review Act (CRA, 5 U.S.C. 801-808).

The CRA requires federal agencies to submit all of their final rules to both houses of Congress and the Government Accountability Office before they can take effect. The act requires that the effective date of "major" rules (e.g., those with at least a $100 million annual effect on the economy) be delayed for 60 calendar days after the date they are submitted to Congress or published in the Federal Register, whichever is later. Although this provision was intended to give Congress an opportunity to disapprove these major rules before they take effect, Congress can use the CRA to disapprove rules even after they have taken effect.

Section 802(a) of the CRA states that a Member of Congress can introduce a resolution of disapproval for any rule starting on the date that the rule is submitted to Congress, and ending no more than 60 "days of continuous session" after that date (i.e., excluding calendar days that either House of Congress is adjourned for more than three days). Section 802(e) states that the Senate has 60 "session days" (i.e., counting only days on which the Senate is in session) from the date the rule is submitted or published in the Federal Register to use expedited procedures to disapprove the rule. However, Section 801(d) of the CRA states that if Congress adjourns its annual session *sine die*[18] less than 60 "legislative days" (in the House of Representatives) or "session days" (in the Senate) after a rule is submitted to it, then the rule is carried over to the next session of Congress and treated as if it was submitted on the 15th legislative or session day of that session of Congress. At that point, the Members have a fresh 60 "days of continuous session" to introduce resolutions of disapproval.[19]

Diseases Not Associated with Exposure to Certain Herbicide Agents

The Agent Orange Act of 1991 (P.L. 102-4) also mandated the VA to publish a notice when the VA determines that a presumption of service connection is not warranted. On June 8, 2010, based on the 2006 IOM report on Agent Orange, the VA issued a notice that a presumption of service connection is *not* warranted based on exposure to herbicides used in Vietnam during the Vietnam Era for the following medical conditions: cancers of the oral cavity (including lips and tongue), pharynx (including tonsils), or nasal cavity (including ears and sinuses); cancers of the pleura, mediastinum, and other unspecified sites within the respiratory system and intrathoracic organs; esophageal cancer; stomach cancer; colorectal cancer (including small intestine and anus); hepatobiliary cancers (liver, gallbladder and bile ducts); pancreatic cancer; bone and joint cancer; melanoma; non-melanoma skin cancer (basal cell and squamous cell); breast cancer; cancers of reproductive organs (cervix, uterus, ovary, testes, and penis; excluding prostate); urinary bladder cancer; renal cancer; cancers of brain and nervous system (including eye); endocrine cancers (thyroid, thymus, and other endocrine); leukemia (other than chronic lymphocytic leukemia (CLL) and B-cell leukemias such as hairy cell lukemia); cancers at other and unspecified sites; neurobehavioral disorders (cognitive and neuropsychiatric); movement disorders (other than amyotrophic lateral sclerosis (ALS) and Parkinson's disease; chronic peripheral nervous system disorders; respiratory disorders; gastrointestinal, metabolic, and digestive disorders (changes in liver enzymes, lipid abnormalities, and ulcers); immune system disorders (immune suppression, allergy, and autoimmunity); circulatory disorders (including hypertension); endometriosis; effects on thyroid homeostasis; certain reproductive effects, i.e., infertility, spontaneous abortion, neonatal or infant death and stillbirth in offspring of exposed people, low birth weight in offspring of exposed people, birth defects (other than spina bifida) in offspring of exposed people, childhood cancer (including acute myelogenous leukemia) in offspring of exposed people; and any other condition for which the VA has not specifically determined a presumption of service connection is warranted.[20]

Children of Vietnam-Era Veterans

Spina Bifida Health Care Program

Vietnam veterans'(both male and female Vietnam veterans) children with the birth defect spina bifida are eligible to receive health care services through the VA (also see "Herbicide Exposure and Veterans Service in Korea").[21] For the purposes of this program spina bifida is defined as all forms or manifestations of spina bifida (except spina bifida occulta). To be eligible to receive health care, the beneficiary must be eligible to receive a monthly monetary allowance. The VA assumes full responsibility for the cost of medical services for the treatment of spina bifida beneficiaries' care, and VA directly reimburses the providers. Generally, care is provided in the private sector, and in some instances, services may also be obtained from VA health care facilities on a space available basis.

The Veterans' Mental Health and Other Care Improvements Act of 2008 (P.L. 110-387) authorized the VA to furnish comprehensive health care services to beneficiaries born with spina bifida. Prior to the enactment of P.L. 110-387, health care services to children born with spina bifida were limited to only health care that was needed to treat spina bifida and associated conditions. This program now covers comprehensive health care that is considered medically necessary and appropriate.

The Children of Women Vietnam Veterans (CWVV) Health Care Program

The Veterans Benefits and Health Care Improvement Act of 2000 (P.L. 106-419) authorized benefits and services for children with certain birth defects who were born to female Vietnam veterans.[22] However, if a birth defect is determined to be familial in a particular family, is a birth-related injury, or is a fetal or neonatal infirmity with well-established causes, it will not be a covered birth defect.

The Agent Orange Registry

The Agent Orange Registry was established in 1978 by the VA for Vietnam veterans concerned about the health effects of exposure to Agent Orange. A veteran choosing to register is eligible for an examination consisting of a medical history, a physical examination, and a series of laboratory tests. Each veteran is also required to answer a set of questions relevant to exposure. In September 2000, the Agent Orange Registry was expanded to include veterans who served in Korea in 1968 and 1969. Since August 2001, the registry is accessible to all U.S. veterans potentially exposed to dioxin or other toxic substances used in herbicides while engaged in military activity. Participating in the registry does not give exposed military personnel automatic access to health and disability compensation benefits. As of March 2010, more than 559,000 veterans have participated in the registry.[23]

Non-Vietnam Veterans Exposed to Agent Orange

Under current law, only Vietnam veterans who served in-country are eligible to receive health care benefits and compensation for service “in Vietnam.”[24] However, under certain circumstances, veterans are eligible for health care and compensation benefits for service outside of Vietnam. A non-Vietnam veteran who claims that an injury or illness resulted from exposure to Agent Orange while serving in the military can apply for service-connected benefits. But unlike Vietnam veterans, non-Vietnam veterans are required to prove they were exposed to Agent Orange. The VA requires the following information in the veteran’s benefit application: a medical diagnosis of a disease or condition the VA recognizes as associated with Agent Orange; evidence of exposure to a chemical contained in the herbicides used in Vietnam; and medical evidence that the disease began or manifested within the designated time frame, if any, for that disease.[25] The DOD has also published a list of areas outside of Vietnam where Agent Orange was used as well as a list of specific areas within the continental U.S. and U.S. territories.[26]

Herbicide Exposure and Veterans Service in Korea

In 2003, Congress passed the Veterans Benefits Act of 2003 (P.L. 108-183).[27] Among other things, section 102 of the Act expanded benefits (health care, monetary allowance, vocational training, and education) for children born with spina bifida of certain veterans who served in Korea.[28] To be eligible for benefits, the veteran must have served in the active military, naval, or air service in or near the Korean Demilitarized Zone (DMZ) between September 1, 1967, and August 31, 1971. Furthermore, even if a veteran served in or near the DMZ within the specified time period, P.L. 108-183 requires the VA in consultation with the DOD to determine whether the veteran was exposed to herbicides during such service. [29]

However, current law does not establish a presumption of herbicide exposure based on service in or near the Korean DMZ. In July 2009, the VA proposed regulations to establish a presumption of exposure to herbicide to any veteran who served between April 1968 and July 1969 in a unit determined by the VA and the DOD to have operated in an area in or near the Korean DMZ in which herbicides were applied.[30] However, according to the proposed regulations, if a veteran served in or near the Korean DMZ during the period between September 1, 1967, and August 31, 1971, but not within the time periods (April 1968 and July 1969) and geographic locations that would qualify for a presumption of exposure under this proposed rule, such service would qualify for benefits only if the VA determines that the veteran was actually exposed to herbicides during such service.[31]

HAAS V. PEAKE[32] (PREVIOUSLY HAAS V. NICHOLSON)[33]

Haas v. Nicholson

On August 16, 2006, the U.S. Court of Appeals for Veterans Claims (CAVC) determined that the veterans who had served in the waters off Vietnam (this class of veterans is generally known as "blue water" veterans) were entitled to a presumption of exposure to Agent Orange.[34] Prior to this CAVC decision,[35] the VA's interpretation of 38 CFR 3.307(a)(6)(iii) was that a service member had to have actually set foot on Vietnamese soil or served on a craft in its rivers (also known as "brown water" veterans) in order to be entitled to the presumption of exposure to Agent Orange. The CAVC specifically held the following: (1) the reference to service "in Vietnam" as used in the statute was ambiguous because there are many definitions of the territory of a nation, and (2) the VA's regulation defining Vietnam service for purposes of granting the presumption of exposure to herbicides, 38 CFR 3.307(a)(6)(iii), was ambiguous when viewed together with 38 CFR 3.313, which also defines service in Vietnam. Because the CAVC determined that ambiguity was present, it also examined the VA's Adjudication Procedure Manual M21-1 (the M21-1 manual)[36] provision from 1991, which stated that the receipt of a Vietnam Service Medal (VSM) would be considered proof of Vietnam service in the absence of "contradictory evidence." In 2002, the VA issued a new M21-1 provision advising VA benefit adjudicators that the receipt of the VSM could indicate service on land in Vietnam but, by itself, was not proof of service in Vietnam because a veteran may have received this medal for service in locations other than Vietnam.[37] The CAVC determined the M21-1 provision to be a substantive rule establishing entitlement to the presumption of exposure to herbicides, and held that the VA's "attempted rescissions" of that M21-1 provision were void because they failed to comply with the notice and comment requirements of the Administrative Procedures Act (APA).[38]

Subsequent Actions

On September 21, 2006, Secretary Nicholson issued a memorandum directing the Board of Veterans Appeals (BVA) to withhold adjudicating all service-connected claims based on exposure to herbicides in which the only evidence of exposure is the receipt of the Vietnam

Service Medal or service on a vessel off the shore of Vietnam.[39] On December 11, 2006, the VA issued a memorandum to its regional offices, instructing them that claims related to *Haas v. Nicholson* should not be adjudicated until the litigation is resolved. As a result, at this time, the BVA has suspended action on *Haas v. Nicholson* claims.[40]

The VA appealed the CAVC decision to the U.S. Court of Appeals for the Federal Circuit in Washington, D.C. Oral argument was held on November 7, 2007.

On November 27, 2007, the VA published a *Federal Register* notice proposing to rescind provisions of its Adjudication Procedures Manual, M21-1 (M21-1), that were found by the CAVC not to have been properly rescinded under the APA.[41] This action was taken by the VA as a preemptive measure in the event the Department did not prevail on appeal in *Haas v. Nicholson*.

Haas v. Peake

Haas v. Peake is the case name on appeal of the previously discussed *Haas v. Nicholson*. On May 8, 2008, the U.S. Court of Appeals for the Federal Circuit ("court") issued a decision reversing the prior CAVC ruling. The court concluded that the VA's interpretation of "service in Vietnam" as requiring the servicemember's presence at some point on the landmass or the inland waters of Vietnam was based on a permissible construction of the statute.[42] The court also stated in its opinion that "Mr. Haas is free to pursue his claim that he was actually exposed to herbicides while on board his ship as it traveled near the Vietnamese coast."[43] However, according to the court's opinion, he is not entitled to the benefit of a presumption related to Agent Orange exposure.[44]

On June 23, 2008, the attorneys for Haas filed a petition with the court for a panel rehearing or a rehearing en banc (that is, the whole panel of judges of the court).[45] On October 9, 2008, the court denied the petition for rehearing.[46] Following this action, Haas petitioned the U.S. Supreme Court for certiorari.[47] On January 21, 2009, the Supreme Court denied the petition for writ of certiorari.[48]

Subsequent Actions

There was a subsequent related proceeding, *Haas v. Shinseki*,[49] on remand from the U.S. Court of Appeals for the Federal Circuit ("the court"), which involved the same plaintiff and the same factual situation. On March 10, 2009, the court vacated the BVA's decision and remanded the claim for further proceedings with the BVA. The effect of this decision is that the veteran was given an opportunity to prove his claim to service-connected benefits for his condition, on the basis of medical and factual evidence.[50] The BVA will reexamine the case and determine whether Haas has a compensable service-connected disability, based on the medical and evidentiary records that Haas presents.

Blue Water Navy Vietnam Veterans and Agent Orange Exposure Study

In late 2009, the VA asked the IOM to conduct a study and prepare a report on whether Vietnam veterans who served in the waters off Vietnam (so-called "blue water" navy veterans) experienced a comparable range of exposures to Agent Orange as the veterans who served on boats or ships that operated on the inland waterways and delta areas of Vietnam ("brown water" navy veterans), and those on the ground in Vietnam. The IOM report is expected to be released sometime in 2011.[51]

Proposed Legislation to Clarify Service in Vietnam

Representative Bob Filner, the Chairman of the House Veterans' Affairs Committee, has introduced the Agent Orange Equity Act of 2009 (H.R. 2254). This legislation, if enacted, would clarify service in Vietnam to include inland waterways, the waters offshore, and airspace above Vietnam during the period beginning on January 9, 1962, and ending on May 7, 1975. Under H.R. 2254, those who have been awarded the Vietnam Service Medal or the Vietnam Campaign Medal and those veterans who served on Johnston Island during the period beginning on April 1, 1972, and ending on September 30, 1977, would also be eligible for disability compensation based on presumptive disease conditions relating to exposure to Agent Orange.

Epidemiologic Research on Vietnam Veterans

Because of the controversy surrounding the use of herbicides in Vietnam, significant research on the health effects of Agent Orange and dioxin exposure has occurred over the last 30 years. The majority of studies have focused on morbidity and mortality of Vietnam veterans and are conducted by the VA, the Centers for Disease Control and Prevention (CDC), the U.S. Air Force, and the various veteran service organizations (VSOs). Despite the abundance of research completed, epidemiologic studies on Agent Orange are historically burdened by the lack of reliable exposure data. The lack of accurate data remains a continued source of frustration for researchers, government officials, and Vietnam-era veterans seeking conclusive information on the health risks of exposure to Agent Orange. Below is a brief description of epidemiologic research conducted by the various agencies.

Centers for Disease Control and Prevention

In 1979, the VA was authorized to conduct an epidemiologic study to determine the association between Agent Orange and the medical concerns of Vietnam-era veterans. In carrying out the congressional mandate, the VA was faced with substantial challenges in determining study design and research protocol, and in 1982, responsibility for the research was transferred from the VA to the CDC. The CDC also faced its own obstacles in research design and were delayed by the lack of exposure data. In response to the difficulty in obtaining exposure data, the CDC attempted an Agent Orange Validation Study to see if indirect estimates of exposure from military records and self-reports could be compared to dioxin serum levels in veterans as a method of determining true exposure. After investigation, the CDC reported that military records and self-reports obtained from the Agent Orange Validation Study were inadequate for identifying the exposed individuals necessary for a large epidemiologic study of dioxin effects. Secondary to the problems faced by the VA and the CDC, a group of government panels and advisory boards determined that the congressionally mandated Agent Orange Study was improbable, and the CDC investigation ended.[52]

Air Force Health Study (AFHS)

Operation Ranch Hand was responsible for spraying herbicides in Vietnam between 1962 and 1971. In 1982, Air Force investigators began a study investigating the long-term health problems of pilots and ground crews engaged in spraying herbicides in Vietnam. The study cohort consisted of more than 1,200 Ranch Hand (the unit responsible for aerially spraying herbicides in Vietnam) veterans and more than 19,000 comparison Air Force veterans who did not spray herbicides. AFHS data collected between 1979 and 1993 revealed no statistically significant differences between the Ranch Hand personnel and the comparison cohort both for all-cause mortality and for cause-specific mortality. The exception was an increased mortality rate for circulatory diseases seen in enlisted ground crew personnel, a group at higher risk for skin exposure to herbicides. In 2005, an AFHS update reviewing 20 years of epidemiologic data on mortality rates reported a small, but significant, increase in all-cause death rates for Ranch Hand veterans.[53] After 20 years of analysis, data collection, and review, a recent IOM publication indicated that diabetes presented as the most serious health problem observed in the AFHS. Type II diabetes was added to the list of service-connected diseases for Vietnam veterans exposed to Agent Orange in 2001.[54] The long-standing AFHS ended on September 30, 2006.

Section 714 of the John Warner National Defense Authorization Act, 2007 (P.L. 109-364), required the Secretary of the Air Force to transfer custody of the AFHS data to the Medical Follow-Up Agency (an agency under the IOM's Board of Military and Veterans Health). This decision to retain the AFHS materials was based on the scientific merit of maintaining herbicide exposure records as a valuable source of medical and epidemiologic data as recommended by the IOM study.[55] Furthermore, P.L. 109-364 required the Secretary of Defense to make $850,000 available to the Air Force in preparation for the transfer of study data to the IOM. An additional $200,000 was to be reimbursed from the DOD to the IOM for costs related to the transfer of study materials from the Air Force.[56]

The Veterans' Benefits Improvement Act of 2008 (P.L. 110-389) authorized the Medical Follow-Up Agency at its discretion to conduct additional research on the assets transferred to the Agency from the AFHS. The Veterans' Benefits Improvement Act of 2008 also authorized $1.2 million for each fiscal year for the maintenance, management, and operation of the assets transferred, and $250,000 for each fiscal year for the conduct of additional research. These activities would be funded by the VA and are authorized through September 30, 2012. Moreover, P.L. 110-389 requires the Medical Follow-Up Agency to submit a report to Congress assessing the feasibility and advisability of conducting additional research on the AFHS after September 30, 2012.

End Notes

[1] U.S. General Accounting Office, *Ground Troops in South Vietnam Were in Areas Sprayed with Herbicide Orange*, GAO 80-23, November 1979, p. 1.

[2] For a more in-depth discussion of the legislative history related to Agent Orange see CRS Report R41405, *Veterans Affairs: Presumptive Service Connection and Disability Compensation*, coordinated by Sidath Viranga Panangala.

[3] The term "service-connected" means, with respect to disability, that such disability was incurred or aggravated in the line of duty in the active military, naval, or air service (38 U.S.C. § 101). VA determines whether veterans have service-connected disabilities and, for those with such disabilities, assigns ratings from 0% to 100% based on the severity of the disability. Percentages are assigned in increments of 10%.

[4] "Limited/suggestive" evidence of no association is when several adequate studies, covering the full range of levels of exposure that human beings are known to encounter, are consistent in not showing a positive association between any magnitude of exposure to herbicides and the outcome of disease.

[5] For detailed information on eligibility for VA health care, see CRS Report R41343, *Veterans Medical Care:FY2011 Appropriations*, by Sidath Viranga Panangala.

[6] 38 C.F.R. § 3.307. The other methods of establishing service connection include through direct service connection—that is, the facts, shown by evidence, establish that a particular injury or disease resulting in a disability was incurred while in service in the Armed Forces (38 C.F.R. § 3.303); through aggravation during service—that is, a preexisting injury or disease will be considered to have been aggravated while in service in the Armed Forces (38 C.F.R. § 3.306); through proximity—that is, a disability, which is proximately due to, or the result of a service-connected disease or injury which is considered to be service-connected (38 C.F.R. § 3.310). For example, a veteran developing cardiovascular disease due to a service-connected amputation of a lower limb; and through a finding, the disability was caused by medical care or vocational rehabilitation provided by the VA—disabilities caused by VA provided medical care or vocational rehabilitation are treated as if they are service-connected (38 U.S.C. § 1151).

[7] For a detailed discussion of presumption of service connection, see CRS Report R41405, *Veterans Affairs: Presumptive Service Connection and Disability Compensation*, coordinated by Sidath Viranga Panangala.

[8] This comprehensive review by the IOM has been repeated at least every two years since 1994 and is authorized to continue until October 2014. *Veterans and Agent Orange* weighs the strengths and limitations of the complete body of epidemiologic evidence on herbicide exposure and manifestation of certain health outcomes. This review then assigns the investigated medical conditions to one of four categories ranging from "sufficient evidence of an association" to "limited or suggestive evidence of no association." For example, in the 2008 *Veterans and Agent Orange* update, this information is available in Table S-1. The latest update was compiled in 2008 and released in July 2009, available at http://www.nap.edu/.

[9] For a detailed discussion of the process for establishing presumption of service connection see CRS Report R41405, *Veterans Affairs: Presumptive Service Connection and Disability Compensation*, coordinated by Sidath Viranga Panangala.

[10] 38.C.F.R. § 3.309(e). In 2003, based on the 2002 update of the IOM report *Veterans and Agent Orange*, the VA issued a regulation designating chronic lymphocytic leukemia ("CLL") and other medical conditions as diseases associated with dioxin. CLL was therefore to be considered "service connected." However, the VA did not re-adjudicate prior claims for CLL, nor did it pay retroactive benefits, arguing that compensation was not applicable to diseases determined to be service-connected after September 20, 2002, the original sunset date of the Agent Orange Act of 1991. Following extensive litigation, the U.S. Court of Appeals for the Ninth Circuit (*Nehmer v. VA,* 494 F.3d 846 (9th Cir. Cal. 2007)) affirmed the district court decision (Nehmer v. VA, 32 F.Supp. 2d 1175 (N.D. Cal. 1999)) and, in effect, confirmed that the VA was obligated to pay disability benefits to all "Agent Orange" veterans with CLL, including those diagnosed after September 20, 2002.

[11] Department of Veterans Affairs, "Presumption of Service Connection for Amyotrophic Lateral Sclerosis," 73 *Federal Register* 54691-54693, September 23, 2008. It should be noted that this presumptive condition is *not* limited to veterans who were potentially exposed to Agent Orange. To be eligible for this presumptive service connection, a veteran must have served on continuous active duty for a period of 90 days or more.

[12] Department of Veterans Affairs, "Presumptive Service Connection for Disease Associated With Exposure to Certain Herbicide Agents: AL Amyloidosis," 74 *Federal Register* 21258-21260, May 7, 2009.

[13] National Academy of Sciences, Institute of Medicine, Veterans and Agent Orange: Update 2008, Washington, DC, 2009.

[14] Department of Veterans Affairs, "VA Extends 'Agent Orange' Benefits to More Veterans, Parkinson's Disease Two Other Illnesses Recognized," press release, October 13, 2009.

[15] Department of Veterans Affairs, "Diseases Associated With Exposure to Certain Herbicide Agents (Hairy Cell Leukemia and Other Chronic B Cell Leukemias, Parkinson's Disease and Ischemic Heart Disease)," 75 Federal Register 14391-14401, March 25, 2010.

[16] Department of Veterans Affairs, "Diseases Associated With Exposure to Certain Herbicide Agents (Hairy Cell Leukemia and Other Chronic B-Cell Leukemias, Parkinson's Disease and Ischemic Heart Disease)," 75 *Federal Register* 53202-53216, August 31, 2010.

[17] Curtis W. Copeland, Specialist in American National Government, made contributions to this section.

[18] The Latin phrase, literally translated as "without day," is used to mean that Congress has adjourned without setting a day for its next meeting. An adjournment sine die, therefore, means that Congress is not scheduled to meet again until the day set by the Constitution (or by law) for its next session to convene.

[19] For more information, see CRS Report RL34633, *Congressional Review Act: Disapproval of Rules in a Subsequent Session of Congress*, by Curtis W. Copeland and Richard S. Beth.

[20] U.S. Department of Veterans Affairs, "Health Effects Not Associated With Exposure to Certain Herbicide Agents." 75 *Federal Register* 32540-32553, June 8, 2010.

[21] A birth child of a Vietnam veteran, regardless of age or marital status, who was conceived after the date on which the Vietnam veteran first entered the Republic of Vietnam, during the period beginning January 9, 1962, and ending May 7, 1975, or a birth child of a Korea veteran, regardless of age or marital status, who was conceived after the date on which the Korea veteran first served in or near the Korean demilitarized zone, during the period beginning September 1, 1967, and ending August 31, 1971.

[22] Covered birth defects include but are not limited to the following: (1) Achondroplasia; (2) Cleft lip and cleft palate; (3) Congenital heart disease; (4) Congenital talipes equinovarus (clubfoot); (5) Esophageal and intestinal atresia; (6) Hallerman-Streiff syndrome; (7) Hip dysplasia; (8) Hirschprung's disease (congenital megacolon); (9) Hydrocephalus due to aqueductal stenosis; (10) Hypospadias; (11) Imperforate anus; (12) Neural tube defects (including spina bifida, encephalocele, and anencephaly); (13) Poland syndrome; (14) Pyloric stenosis; (15) Syndactyly (fused digits); (16) Tracheoesophageal fistula; (17) Undescended testicle; and (18) Williams syndrome (38 C.F.R. § 3.815).

[23] There were a total of 502,056 initial examinations, and 57,353 follow-up examinations; see, http://www.publichealth.va.gov/docs/agentorange/reviews/agentorange-newsletter-jul10.pdf.

[24] Service in the Republic of Vietnam includes service in the waters offshore and services in other locations if conditions of service involved duty or visitation in the Republic of Vietnam.(38 C.F.R. §3.313(a); 38 C.F.R. 3.307(a)(6)(iii)).

[25] If a veteran did not serve in the Republic of Vietnam, but was exposed to an herbicide agent defined in 38 C.F.R. 3.307(a)(6) during active military service, has a disease on the list of diseases subject to presumptive service connection, VA will presume that the disease is due to the exposure to herbicides. Additional information on benefits and compensation for veterans exposed to Agent Orange is available at the U.S. Department of Veterans Affairs, "VA's Guide on Agent Orange Claims, Compensation and Pension Service," updated April 27, 2004, pp. 1-7, at http://www.vba.va.gov/bln/21/Benefits/Herbicide/AOno3.htm.

[26] For a detailed list of sites within and outside the U.S., see http://www.publichealth.va.gov/exposures/agentorange/outside_vietnam.asp.

[27] P.L. 108-183, among other the bills, contained provisions from H.R. 2297 (H.Rept. 108-211) and S. 1132 (S.Rept. 108-169).

[28] This applies to all forms and manifestations of spina bifida, except spina bifida occulta.

[29] 38 U.S.C. § 1821. Furthermore, the DOD has advised VA that herbicides were not applied within the DMZ, but were applied in some adjacent areas. Specifically, the DOD has reported that herbicides were applied between April 1968 and July 1969 along a strip of land 151 miles long and up to 350 yards wide along the southern edge of the DMZ north of the civilian control line. The herbicide agents were applied through hand spraying and hand distribution of pelletized herbicides. According to the DOD, there was no aerial spraying. The DOD also has provided the VA a list of the military units that are currently known to have operated in that area during the period that herbicides were applied [see U.S. Department of Veterans Affairs, "Herbicide Exposure and Veterans With Covered Service in Korea," 74 Federal Register 36640-36648, July 24, 2009].

[30] U.S. Department of Veterans Affairs, "Herbicide Exposure and Veterans With Covered Service in Korea," 74 Federal Register 36640-36648, July 24, 2009.

[31] Ibid.

[32] 525 F.3d 1168 (Fed. Cir. 2008).

[33] 20 Vet. App. 257 (2006). Jonathan L. Haas was a member of the U.S. Navy Reserve components that served in the waters off Vietnam and received the Vietnam Service Medal (VSM). He claimed that his diabetes mellitus and resulting medical complications were related to his exposure to Agent Orange that drifted offshore, and filed a disability claim with the VA. The VA denied the claim on the grounds that servicemembers had to have actually set foot on Vietnamese soil in order to be eligible for benefits.

[34] For further information on the CAVC, see CRS Report RS22561, *Veterans Affairs: The U.S. Court of Appeals for Veterans Claims—Judicial Review of VA Decision Making*, by Douglas Reid Weimer.

[35] U.S. Court of Appeals for Veterans Claims (CAVC), 20 Vet. App. 257 (2006).

[36] The M21-1 is an internal manual used to provide guidance to VA benefit adjudicators on procedures for adjudicating claims for compensation, pension, dependency and indemnity compensation, accrued benefits, and burial allowance.

[37] The VSM was awarded to all members of the Armed Forces who served between July 3, 1965, and March 28, 1973, either (1) in Vietnam and contiguous waters and airspace thereover, or (2) in Thailand, Laos, or Cambodia, or airspace thereover, in direct support of operations in Vietnam. See http://www.history.navy.mil/medals/vsn.htm.

[38] 5 U.S.C. § 706(2)(A).

[39] Memorandum No. 01-06-24 Subj. Processing of claims for compensation on exposure to herbicides affected by Haas. v. Nicholson-imposition of stay. See http://vets.yuku.com/topic/4439/t/HAAS-v-NICHOLSON-IMPOSITION-OF-STAY.html.

[40] For further details on the BVA, see CRS Report RL33704, *Veterans Affairs: The Appeal Process for Veterans' Claims*, by Douglas Reid Weimer.

[41] Department of Veterans Affairs, "Rescission of Manual M21-1 Provisions Related To Exposure to Herbicides Based on Receipt of the Vietnam Service Medal," 72 Federal Register 66218-66219, November 27, 2007.

[42] *Haas v. Peake,* 525 F.3d 1168 (Fed. Cir. 2008).

[43] Ibid., p. 1197.

[44] Ibid.

[45] No. 2007-7037.

[46] 544 F.3d 1306 (Fed. Cir. 2008).

[47] 38 U.S.C. § 7292(c). A petition for certiorari is a request for the Supreme Court to review the decision of the lower court. See http://www.techlawjournal.com/glossary/legal/certiorari.htm.

[48] 129 S.Ct. 1002 (2009). This action had the effect of affirming the decision of the Court of Appeals which had previously reversed the decision of the CAVC.

[49] 22 Vet. App. 385; 2009 U.S. App. Vet. Claims LEXIS 315 (2009).

[50] As a result of the various judicial decisions, Haas is not able to use the "agent orange presumption" in proving his claim. Rather, he must prove his claim through factual and medical evidence.

[51] More details about this project is available at http://www8.nationalacademies.org/cp/projectview.aspx?key=49201.

[52] The government panel and advisory groups included the CDC advisory group, the Science Panel of the Domestic Policy Council's Agent Orange Working Group, and the Agent Orange Advisory Panel of the Congressional Office of Technology Assessment.

[53] Norma Ketchum and Joel Michalek, "Postservice Mortality of Air Force Veterans Occupationally Exposed to Herbicides During the Vietnam War: 20-year follow-up results," *Military Medicine*, vol. 170, no. 5 (May 2005), pp. 406-413.

[54] National Academies, Institute of Medicine, *Disposition of the Air Force Health Study*, 2006, p. 55., and see U.S. Department of Veterans Affairs , "Disease Associated With Exposure to Certain Herbicide Agents: Type 2 Diabetes," 66 *Federal Register* 2376, January 11, 2001.

[55] Ibid., p. 4.

[56] U.S. Congress, Conference Committees, *National Defense Authorization Act for Fiscal Year 2007*, a report to accompany H.R. 5122, 109th Congress, 2nd sess., H.Rept. 109-702. *Congressional Record*, daily edition, vol. 152 (September 29, 2006), pp. H8061-H8536.

In: Veterans Benefits
Editors: George B. Meyers and Alice M. Glaskin
ISBN: 978-1-61209-581-3

Chapter 7

VETERANS' BENEFITS: CURRENT LIFE INSURANCE PROGRAMS

Christine Scott

SUMMARY

The Department of Veterans Affairs (VA) administers and supervises several life insurance programs for active servicemembers and veterans. The VA supervises the Servicemembers' Group Life Insurance (SGLI) and Veterans' Group Life Insurance (VGLI) programs, which are administered by the Office of Servicemembers' Group Life Insurance (OSGLI), a division of Prudential Financial. The Service-Disabled Veterans' Insurance (S-DVI) program, on the other hand, is administered entirely by the VA. Access to VA-administered life insurance programs gives servicemembers and veterans, who may not be eligible for private life insurance policies, the opportunity to carry group life insurance. This provides for their families in the event of the servicemember's or veteran's death.

In September 1965, with the passage of P.L. 89-214, Congress established the SGLI program and mandated the VA to enter into an agreement with the private insurance industry to meet the insurance needs of Vietnam era servicemembers. As a result, VA established an agreement with Prudential Financial to administer its policies. When first enacted, the SGLI program provided up to $10,000 in coverage for policyholders. Today, servicemembers can receive a maximum of $400,000 insurance coverage under the program.

On August 1, 1974, with the enactment of P.L. 93-289, VGLI became available to servicemembers. VGLI provides for the conversion of SGLI after separation from active military duty. VGLI is a five-year renewable term policy that, like SGLI, provides a maximum of $400,000 of coverage.

Servicemembers may have their SGLI and VGLI proceeds paid either as a lump sum or over a period of 36 months. Since 1999, if the member chose to have his or her benefits paid as a lump sum without specifying that the payment be made via a single check, beneficiaries would have received payments via retained asset accounts called Alliance Accounts. However, in light of recent media coverage condemning this practice as a violation of contractual agreements, Prudential is to now send beneficiaries of VA life-insurance policies a check when they ask for a lump-sum benefit payment rather than keeping the money in an Alliance Account and mailing a draft book, unless an Alliance Account is specifically requested. Free financial counseling is available to SGLI and VGLI beneficiaries if the policyholder chooses to have payments made via an Alliance Account.

During the Korean War, before SGLI and VGLI were established, Congress passed the Insurance Act of 1951 (P.L. 82-23) and established the S-DVI program. S-DVI was created to meet the insurance needs of certain veterans with service-connected disabilities, many of whom would not be eligible for private life insurance due to their service-connected disabilities. Currently, policies are issued for a maximum face value of $10,000. Retained asset accounts are not offered under the S-DVI program.

Several bills have been introduced in the 111th Congress that would affect the VA's current life insurance programs: H.R. 5993, H.R. 2713, H.R. 1037, S. 3718, and S. 728.

This chapter provides information on the current VA life insurance programs available for servicemembers and veterans, management and administration issues, and associated policy issues and legislation.

INTRODUCTION

The Department of Veterans Affairs (VA) has administered and supervised several life insurance programs for servicemembers and veterans since 1919. Currently, three VA life insurance programs that provide benefits to the families of servicemembers and veterans are still enrolling new policyholders. These programs are Servicemembers' Group Life Insurance (SGLI), Veterans' Group Life Insurance (VGLI), and Service-Disabled Veterans' Insurance (S-DVI). The VA's Regional Office and Insurance Center (VAROIC) in Philadelphia, PA, supervises SGLI and VGLI, but the day-to-day administration of the programs is handled by the Office of Servicemembers' Group Life Insurance (OSGLI), a division of the Prudential Insurance Company of America. The Service-Disabled Veterans' Insurance (S-DVI) program, on the other hand, is administered entirely by the VA. Access to VA-administered life insurance programs gives servicemembers and veterans, who may not be eligible for private life insurance policies, the opportunity to carry group life insurance. This provides for their families in the event of the servicemember's or veteran's death.

The VA agreed in September 2009 to allow Prudential Financial to provide payments of lump-sum benefits through Prudential's Alliance Accounts (a retained asset account) unless the beneficiary elects a single check.[1] Recent media coverage on the issue has caused the VA to revamp its claims materials, to create more transparency for SGLI and VGLI beneficiaries, and to require payments of lump-sum benefits through a single check unless the beneficiary elects to use an Alliance Account.[2] Additionally, concerns have been raised about the limited amount of coverage offered to S-DVI policyholders, which is capped at $10,000.

This chapter is structured into three major sections. The first section provides an overview of the VA's different life insurance programs, including eligibility requirements, premium rates, and benefits. The second section describes the VA's management and administrative structure as well as how policy proceeds to beneficiaries are currently paid out for SGLI, VGLI, and S-DVI. The third section of the report discusses major areas of congressional interest and policy issues as they pertain to SGLI, VGLI, and S-DVI.

SERVICEMEMBERS' GROUP LIFE INSURANCE PROGRAM

In September 1965, Congress established the Servicemembers' Group Life Insurance (SGLI) program (P.L. 89-214) by mandating the VA to enter into an agreement with the private insurance industry to meet the insurance needs of Vietnam era servicemembers.[3] Since 1965, Congress has amended SGLI to include all eligible servicemembers in the uniformed service.

The SGLI program, through a group policy issued by the Prudential Insurance Company of America, provides low-cost term insurance protection to servicemembers. It is administered by the Department of Veterans Affairs Regional Office and Insurance Center's (VAROIC's) Office of Servicemembers' Group Life Insurance (OSGLI) located in Philadelphia, PA. When first enacted, the SGLI program provided up to $10,000 coverage for members. Today, all servicemembers can receive a maximum of $400,000 insurance coverage under the program. As of January 2010, about 2,402,500 members of the uniformed service were covered under the program.[4]

Under the Veterans' Survivor Benefits Improvement Act of 2001 (P.L. 107-14), Congress extended coverage to the spouses and children of servicemembers covered under the SGLI program. The FY2005 Emergency Supplemental Appropriations Act for Defense, the Global War on Terror, and Tsunami Relief (P.L. 109-13) added Traumatic Injury Protection Insurance to SGLI, which extended the program to provide short-term financial assistance to servicemembers suffering from traumatic injuries.[5]

Eligibility Requirements for SGLI

Full-time and part-time life insurance coverage are both provided through the SGLI program.[6] According to the *Servicemembers' and Veterans' Group Life Insurance Handbook*, full-time coverage is provided to the following **active duty servicemembers** under calls or orders that exceed 30 days:

- commissioned, warrant, and enlisted members of the Army, Navy, Air Force, Marine Corps, Coast Guard, National Oceanic and Atmospheric Administration (NOAA) Commissioned Corps, and Public Health Service (PHS) Commissioned Corps;
- members of a uniformed service's Ready Reserve/National Guard that are assigned to a unit or position in which they may be required to perform active duty or active duty for training and are scheduled to perform at least 12 periods of inactive duty training annually that is creditable for retirement purpose under Title 10 of the *U.S. Code*;[7]
- members of the Individual Ready Reserve (IRR) who volunteer for assignment to a "mobilization" category under Sec. 12304 (i)(1) of Title 10 of the *U.S. Code*;

- cadets or midshipmen of the U.S. Military Academy, U.S. Naval Academy, U.S. Air Force Academy, and the U.S. Coast Guard Academy; and
- Reserve Officers' Training Corps (ROTC) members, cadets, or midshipmen while attending field training or practice cruises.[8]

The following members of the **Reserves** (who are ineligible for full-time coverage) are eligible for part-time coverage while on active duty under calls or orders that exceed 30 days:

- commissioned, warrant, and enlisted members of the Army, Navy, Air Force, Marine Corps, and Coast Guard Reserves (except temporary members of the Coast Guard Reserve);
- members of the IRR during one-day call-ups;
- PHS Reserve Corps;
- Army National Guard and Air National Guard while performing duty under Sections 316, 502, 503, 504, or 505 of Title 32 of the *U.S. Code*;[9] and
- ROTC members, cadets, and midshipmen while attending field training or practice cruises.[10]

SGLI Coverage and Premium Rates

Currently, the maximum SGLI coverage is $400,000.[11] This coverage amount ($400,000) is automatic when the servicemember enters into a period of active duty or reserve status and can be elected in $50,000 decrements from the maximum amount. Members may elect to either decline coverage or reduce coverage by completing SGLI program Form SGLV-8286.[12] However, proof of good health is required[13] if the member decides to obtain or increase coverage after he or she had previously chosen to reduce or decline coverage.[14]

This insurance is forfeited when an insured servicemember is found guilty of mutiny, treason, spying, desertion, or, as a conscientious objector, refuses to perform service or refuses to wear his or her uniform.[15]

Full-time Coverage

Servicemembers who are eligible for full-time SGLI coverage are covered through their period of active duty or qualifying reserve status. They are also covered for a period of 120 days (with no premium) after their separation or release from active duty or reserve status.[16]

The Veterans' Housing Opportunity and Benefits Improvement Act of 2006 (P.L. 109-233) extended the free 120-day coverage period to two years for certain disabled servicemembers and their dependents. This change allows SGLI policyholders that are totally disabled (unable to work) at the time of their separation or release from service to keep their SGLI coverage for up to two years. This coverage is classified as the SGLI Disability Extension, and the member is obligated to apply for the coverage after he or she has separated from service.[17]

When a servicemember with full-time SGLI coverage is released from active duty or the Reserves, he or she may convert his or her coverage to VGLI or to a commercial life insurance policy with any of the 38 participating commercial insurance companies.[18]

Table 1. Monthly SGLI Premiums

Amount of Insurance	Monthly SGLI Premium
$50,000	$3.25
$100,000	$6.50
$150,000	$9.75
$200,000	$13.00
$250,000	$16.25
$300,000	$19.50
$350,000	$22.75
$400,000	$26.00

Source: Department of Veterans Affairs, Regional Office and Insurance Center, *VA Life Insurance Programs for Veterans and Servicemembers,* Philadelphia, PA, January 2010.

Note: These premiums do not include the $1.00 premium for Traumatic Servicemembers' Group Life Insurance (TSGLI) coverage. Full-time servicemembers are charged one of the above premiums once monthly. Part-time servicemembers are charged one of the above premiums once annually.

Part-time Coverage

Servicemembers eligible for part-time SGLI coverage are only covered during the time in which they are on active duty or active duty for training, and the period in which they are traveling to and from such duty. Part-time coverage members are eligible for the free 120-day period of coverage only if they incur a disability or a preexisting disability is aggravated during a period of duty.[19]

Beneficiaries

Servicemembers can select anyone as the beneficiary of their insurance policies. If a member fails to name someone, the insurance proceeds, by law, must be distributed in the following order:

1. widow or widower, or, if none,
2. children (not including stepchildren), or, if none,
3. parents, or, if none,
4. executor of the estate, or, if none,
5. other next of kin.[20]

If the servicemember chooses not to be insured under the SGLI program, chooses to be insured for less than the SGLI maximum amount, or names someone other than his or her spouse or child as the beneficiary, the law requires that the spouse of the servicemember must be notified by the uniformed service.[21]

Premium Rates

The cost of SGLI is generally shared by the servicemember and the government. Each servicemember is responsible for paying a monthly premium (unless in a combat zone, in which case the government pays the full premium), and the government pays the cost of all death claims. The SGLI insurance premium is deducted from the servicemember's pay. The premium rates are mutually agreed upon by the VA and the contractor (Prudential Insurance Company of America).

Currently, the basic SGLI premium rate decreased from the 2007 rate of 7.0 cents per month per $1,000 of coverage, to 6.5 cents per month per $1,000 of coverage.[22] **Table 1** shows premium rates for both full-time and part-time active duty servicemembers and reservists:[23]

Extra Hazard of Duty Cost

Each branch of service is liable, under law, to pay the additional cost of claims due to the extra hazards of serving in the military.[24] In 2009, extra hazard costs amounted to $213 million. This amount is determined by the VA and paid by the Department of Defense (DOD) on behalf of the uniformed service.[25]

Each year the VA actuaries study the mortality rate of the most recent three years of servicemembers' claim experience. This allows them to develop the average death rate by age. The rate is used to determine the expected number of death claims. At the end of each policy year, the expected death claims are compared with the actual number of incurred death claims. If the actual death claims exceed the estimated death claims, the excess claims are multiplied by the average amount of insurance per member to determine the extra hazard cost for each uniformed service.

Table 2. Monthly Premium Rates for SGLI Spousal Coverage

	Age of Spouse						
Amount of Insurance	**Under Age 35**	**Age 35 to 39**	**Age 40 to 44**	**Age 45 to 49**	**Age 50 to 54**	**Age 55 to 59**	**Age 60 and Over**
$100,000	5.50	7.00	9.00	14.00	27.00	40.00	52.00
$90,000	4.95	6.30	8.10	12.60	24.30	36.00	46.80
$80,000	4.40	5.60	7.20	11.20	21.60	32.00	41.60
$70,000	3.85	4.90	6.30	9.80	18.90	28.00	36.40
$60,000	3.30	4.20	5.40	8.40	16.20	24.00	31.40
$50,000	2.75	3.50	4.50	7.00	13.50	20.00	26.00
$40,000	2.20	2.80	3.60	5.60	10.80	16.00	20.80
$30,000	1.65	2.10	2.70	4.20	8.10	12.00	15.60
$20,000	1.10	1.40	1.80	2.80	5.40	8.00	10.40
$10,000	0.55	0.70	0.90	1.40	2.70	4.00	5.20

Source: Department of Veterans Affairs, Regional Office and Insurance Center, *VA Life Insurance Programs for Veterans and Servicemembers,* Philadelphia, PA, January 2010.

Notes: Spouses of servicemembers can receive coverage up to $100,000. However, the spouse's coverage amount can never exceed that of the servicemember's coverage amount. For example, if the servicemember has $70,000 of SGLI coverage, the spouse's coverage can be a maximum of $70,000 (Department of Veterans Affairs, Regional Office and Insurance Center, *VA Life Insurance Programs for Veterans and Servicemembers,* Philadelphia, PA, January 2010, p. 36, http://www.insurance.va.gov/gli/glihandbook/glibooklet2010.pdf.

If the annual extra hazard cost paid is lower than the estimated amount, Prudential Insurance will refund the excess funds to the VA. Excess funds are deposited into the revolving fund. If the extra hazard cost paid exceeds the annual estimated amount, then the VA is responsible for reimbursing the insurance company (Prudential) from the revolving fund.[26]

Family Servicemembers' Group Life Insurance Coverage

SGLI coverage was extended to the spouses and dependent children of insured servicemembers by the Veterans' Survivor Benefits Improvements Act of 2001 (P.L. 107-14).

Family Servicemembers' Group Life Insurance (FSGLI) coverage is automatically issued to the member's spouse and children, based on the information in the servicemember's personnel records. Members may decline family coverage or may elect reduced coverage by completing SGLI program Form SGLV-8286A, Family Coverage Election.[27] However, proof of good health of the spouse or child is required if the member decides to obtain or increase coverage for his or her spouse or child after he or she has previously chosen to reduce or decline coverage.[28]

FSGLI Spousal Coverage

Spouses of servicemembers on active duty or reservists, including National Guard members eligible for full-time SGLI coverage, can be insured up to the maximum amount of $100,000 in increments of $10,000. However, spousal coverage cannot exceed the servicemember's SGLI coverage. Premiums for spousal coverage are deducted from the servicemember's or reservist's pay.[29] **Table 2** shows the premium rates for spouses based on age and amount of coverage.[30]

A spouse of a servicemember or active duty reservist may convert his or her coverage to a commercial life insurance policy with any of 38 participating commercial insurance companies. Coverage for a spouse will end 120 days after any of the following events:

- The date the servicemember elects (in writing) to terminate his or her spouse's coverage;
- The date the servicemember elects (in writing) to terminate his or her own SGLI coverage;
- The date of the servicemember's death;
- The date the servicemember separates from service; or
- The date of the servicemember's divorce from his or her spouse.[31]

FSGLI Child Coverage

A child is considered to be a dependent of a servicemember if the child is unmarried and under the age of 18, or became permanently incapable of self-support before the age of 18. Dependent children include all natural born children, legally adopted children, and stepchildren who are under the care of the servicemember. A child is also considered to be a dependent if he or she is between the ages of 18 and 22 and is enrolled in an approved educational institution. Dependent children covered under an active duty servicemember's or reservist's SGLI policy are insured at the maximum amount of $10,000 each (at no cost to the servicemember). The child is covered up to 120 days after the servicemember has separated from service.[32]

The Veterans' Benefits Improvement Act of 2008 (P.L. 110-389) added benefits for families of stillborn children born on or after October 10, 2008, under the FSGLI program. Previously, stillborn children were excluded from coverage. Servicemembers who experience the death of such a dependent child are eligible to receive a $10,000 payment (the maximum amount under FSGLI child coverage).

Coverage for a child will end 120 days after the servicemember's separation or release from service or assignment (in the case of Ready Reserve). There are currently no conversion options for children.

SGLI Traumatic Injury Protection Program

Since its inception in 2005, the Traumatic Servicemembers' Group Life Insurance (TSGLI) program has provided short-term financial assistance to servicemembers who suffer from traumatic injuries while on active duty.[33] TSGLI is an automatic coverage program under the SGLI program, and its purpose is to ease the burden for servicemembers and their families during times of extensive recovery and rehabilitation. In 2008, after an extensive "TSGLI Year-One Review," the VA increased the number of traumatic injuries covered under this program and relaxed the criteria for other injuries.[34]

Eligibility

Servicemembers who are covered under the SGLI program are automatically covered by the TSGLI program. However, TSGLI does not cover spouses and children who are covered under the SGLI program, nor does it cover those under the VGLI program. Eligibility and certification for payment are determined and provided by each member's uniformed service.[35]

Losses covered by TSGLI include the following conditions:

- total and permanent loss of sight, speech, or hearing;
- amputation of hand or the loss of four fingers on the same hand or loss of a thumb;
- amputation of foot or loss of all toes;
- loss of four toes on the same foot or the loss of the big toe;
- limb salvage;
- quadriplegia, paraplegia, hemiplegia, or uniplegia;
- burns (2nd degree or more covering 20% or more of the body or 20% or more of the face);
- facial reconstruction;
- coma resulting from traumatic injury;
- inability to perform two activities of daily living due to traumatic brain injury;[36]
- inability to perform two activities of daily living due to other traumatic injury; and
- continuous 15-day inpatient hospital care due to traumatic injury.[37]

The Veterans' Benefits Act of 2010 (P.L. 111-275) provided that the Secretary may distinguish in payments for qualifying loss of a dominant hand and qualifying loss of a non-dominant hand.

Losses Excluded from TSGLI Payment

Injuries sustained while committing or attempting to commit a felony and losses caused by the following are excluded from TSGLI payment:

- mental disorder;
- mental or physical illness or disease, unless the illness or disease is caused by a pyogenic (pus forming, often from a wound) infection, biological, chemical, or radiological weapon, or accidental ingestion of a contaminated substance;
- attempted suicide;
- self-inflicted wounds;
- diagnostic procedures, preventive medical procedures (i.e., inoculations), medical or surgical treatment for an illness or disease, or any complications arising from such procedures or treatment; or
- the member's willful use of illegal or controlled substances, unless they are administered or taken on the advice of medical professionals.[38]

Benefit Amount

TSGLI benefit amounts depend on the type and severity of a servicemember's injury and range from $25,000 to a maximum of $100,000. Servicemembers who suffered injuries between October 7, 2001, and December 1, 2005, as a result of serving in Operation Enduring Freedom or Operation Iraqi Freedom (whether insured by SGLI or not) may receive retroactive TSGLI benefits.[39]

TSGLI premiums are $1.00 per month and are deducted from the servicemember's pay.[40]

VETERANS' GROUP LIFE INSURANCE PROGRAM

On August 1, 1974, Veterans' Group Life Insurance (VGLI) became available to former servicemembers (P.L. 93-289). VGLI provides for the conversion of SGLI after separation from active duty. The administration of the VGLI program is handled by the OSGLI, a division of the Prudential Insurance Company of America. VGLI is a five-year renewable term policy which provides a maximum of $400,000 of coverage. VGLI policyholders have the right to renew their coverage at the end of each five-year term period. Policyholders may also convert VGLI to an individual commercial policy at any time with any of the 38 participating private companies without proof of insurability.[41] VGLI has no cash, loan, paid up, or extended values and does not pay dividends.

Eligibility Requirements for VGLI

Veterans eligible for the VGLI program are:

- Ready Reserves/National Guard SGLI policyholders who are separated, retired, or released from assignment;
- insured SGLI members who are being released from active duty or active duty for training under a call or order to duty that does not specify a period of less than 31 days;
- Ready Reservists who have part-time SGLI coverage and who, while performing duty (or traveling directly to or from duty), suffer an injury or disability that causes them to be uninsurable at standard premium rates;[42] and
- people assigned to the IRR of a military service or to the Inactive National Guard (ING). This includes members of the Public Health Service Inactive Reserve Corps (IRC).[43]

After separation from service, members have 120 days to apply for VGLI without providing evidence of insurability (good health). Members who do not apply for VGLI within 120 days of separation from service have an additional year in which to apply for VGLI. During this additional year members are required to submit the initial premium and provide evidence of insurability (good health) in addition to the application for VGLI. If a member does not apply for VGLI within the one year and 120 days allotted following separation from service, he or she becomes ineligible for coverage under VGLI.

Members who are totally disabled[44] at the time of separation from active duty and are granted a free two-year extended SGLI coverage period are automatically enrolled in VGLI at the end of the two-year extension period.[45]

Table 3. VGLI Monthly Premium Rates

	Amount of Insurance					
Age	**$400,000**	**$300,000**	**$200,000**	**$100,000**	**$50,000**	**$10,000**
Thru 29	$32.00	$24.00	$16.00	$8.00	$4.00	$0.80
30 thru 34	40.00	30.00	20.00	10.00	5.00	1.00
35 thru 39	52.00	39.00	26.00	13.00	6.50	1.30
40 thru 44	68.00	51.00	34.00	17.00	8.50	1.70
45 thru 49	88.00	66.00	44.00	22.00	11.00	2.20
50 thru 54	144.00	108.00	72.00	36.00	18.00	3.60
55 thru 59	268.00	201.00	134.00	67.00	33.50	6.70
60 thru 64	432.00	324.00	216.00	108.00	54.00	10.80
65 thru 69	600.00	450.00	300.00	150.00	75.00	15.00
70 thru 74	900.00	675.00	450.00	225.00	112.50	22.50
75 & Over	1,800.00	1,350.00	900.00	450.00	225.00	45.00

Source: Department of Veterans Affairs, Regional Office and Insurance Center, *VA Life Insurance Programs for Veterans and Servicemembers*, Philadelphia, PA, January 2010, p. 42, https://www.insurance.va.gov/gli/glihandbook/ glibooklet2010.pdf.

VGLI Coverage and Premium Rates

The maximum amount of coverage for VGLI is $400,000 if the member separated from service after September 1, 2005. If the member separated from service prior to September 1, 2005, his or her maximum coverage is $250,000 (P.L. 109-80). VGLI coverage is issued in multiples of $10,000 up to the maximum amount of coverage. VGLI coverage, at the time of conversion from SGLI, may not exceed the amount of SGLI coverage that the member had at the time he or she was released from active duty or the reserves. However, a member may increase his or her coverage once in every five-year period by $25,000 if the member is under the age of 60, and still to the statutory maximum coverage amount.[46] To be covered under VGLI, members must pay premiums. VGLI premium rates are determined by age and amount of insurance. For example, a member who is aged 29 or younger would pay $32 per month for the maximum $400,000 coverage, while a member who is aged 75 or older would pay $1,800 per month for the same $400,000 coverage.[47] **Table 3** lists monthly premium rates per age group per coverage amount.

VGLI Payment of Premiums

The VGLI program offers various options for paying premiums. Policyholders may choose to pay the premiums on a monthly, quarterly, semi-annual, or annual basis. Discounted premiums are available for some of these options. **Table 4** shows the different payment options available under VGLI and their associated discounts.

Table 4. VGLI Premium Payment Options

Frequency of Premium Payment	Methods of Premium Payment Available	Annual Premium Discount Rate
Monthly	Allotment from military pay	No Discount
	Deduction from VA compensation payments	
	Check	
	On-demand deduction from checking account or credit card account	
Quarterly	Check	2.50% Discount
	On-demand deduction from checking account or credit card account	
Semi-annually	Check	3.75% Discount
	On-demand deduction from checking account or credit card account	
Annually	Check	5.00% Discount
	On-demand deduction from checking account or credit card account	

Source: Department of Veterans Affairs, Regional Office and Insurance Center, *VA Life Insurance Programs for Veterans and Servicemembers*, Philadelphia, PA, January 2010, p. 42, https://www .insurance.va.gov/gli/glihandbook/ glibooklet2010.pdf.

Table 5. VGLI Coverage Reduction Schedule

Age Group	Coverage Level	Monthly Premium
65-69	$150,000	$225
70-74	$100,000	$225
75 & over	$50,000	$225

Source: Department of Veterans Affairs, Regional Office and Insurance Center, *VA Life Insurance Programs for Veterans and Servicemembers*, Philadelphia, PA, January 2010, p. 43, https://www.insurance.va.gov/gli/glihandbook/ glibooklet2010.pdf.

Table 6. S-DVI Current Coverage Information

Number of veterans with 5-year term policies	59,183
Number of veterans with permanent plan policies	115,718
Total amount of insurance in force	$2,053,528,077[a]
Average coverage per veteran	$11,741
Average age of covered veteran	60.5
Average annual death rate	35.5 per 1,000
Total disbursements FY2009	125,321,271
Percentage of policies on premium waivers	46%

Source: Department of Veterans Affairs, Regional Office and Insurance Center, *VA Life Insurance Programs for Veterans and Servicemembers*, Philadelphia, PA, January 2010, p. 26, https://www.insurance.va.gov/gli/glihandbook/ glibooklet2010.pdf.

Note: Veterans may choose either a five-year term policy or a permanent plan policy when applying for S-DVI.

a. This number includes both S-DVI policies with coverage of $10,000 and S-DVI policies with coverage of $30,000 (S-DVI coverage of $10,000 plus Supplemental S-DVI coverage of $20,000).

VGLI Coverage Reduction Schedule

As members age, they incur higher premium rates for insurance coverage, as shown in **Table 5**. To lessen or maintain cost at older ages, members may gradually reduce the amount of their VGLI coverage. VA recommends the following schedule that will allow veterans to maintain level premiums ($225 per month) while reducing coverage at ages 65 and older:

Commercial Conversion Criteria

VGLI policyholders may convert to individual commercial policies at any time with a commercial company that participates in the program without proof of insurability so long as VGLI premiums are paid up to the date of the conversion.[48] However, once a member converts his or her coverage to a commercial policy he or she may no longer renew his or her VGLI coverage. Veterans that convert to commercial policies are issued standard premium rates regardless of their health, but coverage may not exceed the amount of VGLI coverage that the members had at the time of conversion. Additionally, the conversion policy must be a permanent policy, such as a whole life policy. Other types of policies, such as term, variable life, or universal life insurance, are not allowed as conversion policies. Spouses and children may not be covered under VGLI.

In order to convert a VGLI policy, the veteran must:

- Select a company from the participating companies listing;
- Submit an application to the local sales office of the company selected;
- Obtain a letter from the OSGLI verifying coverage; and
- Give a copy of that notice to the agent who takes the application.

SERVICE-DISABLED VETERANS' INSURANCE PROGRAM

During the Korean War, Congress passed the Insurance Act of 1951 (P.L. 82-23) and established the Service-Disabled Veterans' Insurance (S-DVI) program, which is administered entirely by the VA. S-DVI was created to meet the insurance needs of certain veterans with service-connected disabilities, many of whom would not be eligible for private life insurance due to their service-connected disabilities.[49] S-DVI is available as a permanent plan or as a five-year term policy for disabled veterans, and policyholders can apply for up to $10,000 in coverage. Policies for this insurance are issued with the letters "RH" in front of the policy number. RH insurance is considered nonparticipating, which means that no dividends are paid to policyholders. S-DVI is still being issued to new policyholders, and it is currently the only issue of direct VA life insurance for veterans that is open to new policyholders.[50] **Table 6** shows basic statistics related to S-DVI, including the current number of veterans covered and the average age of covered veterans.

Eligibility Requirements for S-DVI ("RH")

To be eligible for S-DVI, a veteran must have

- been released from military service for reasons other than dishonorable discharge or bad conduct discharge awarded at General Court-Martial;[51]
- been released from active duty on or after April 25, 1951;
- been rated for a service-connected disability or disabilities (even if only 0%), but is otherwise in good health; and
- applied within two years of receiving a rating for a new service-connected disability.[52]

Ratings for service-connected disabilities are determined by the severity of the veteran's disability on a scale from 0% to 100%. 0% is a valid rating and is different from no rating at all. A 0% rating means that a service-connected disability exists, but it is not so disabling that it entitles the veteran to compensation payments. Under S-DVI, all veterans with a service-connected disability are eligible for coverage, no matter the rating. However, the veteran must submit an insurance application within two years from the date that he or she is notified about the disability rating. If the veteran does not apply within that time but service connection is later established for some new condition, the veteran will then have two years from the date of notice of that new condition to apply.

S-DVI Premiums and Disability Provisions

Premiums charged for S-DVI coverage are

- based on the rates that healthy people would have been charged when the program started in 1951, and based on 1941 mortality tables; and
- waived for veterans who are totally disabled.

Because the program insures many veterans who have severe disabilities, premium payments are insufficient to pay all claims and are supplemented yearly by congressional appropriations.

Premiums paid for S-DVI coverage increase as policyholders get older. On November 1, 2000, to provide financial relief from high premium rates for veterans at advanced ages, "RH" term premiums were "capped" at the age 70 renewal rate. Therefore, annual premiums for policyholders were "capped" at $69.73 per $1,000 of coverage.[53]

A major issue for "RH" policyholders is that "RH" premiums are much higher than standard commercial rates because they are based on outdated mortality (1941) tables. The following statement was issued by Representative Joe Donnelly, concerning the VA's current use of 1941 mortality tables to determine S-DVI premium rates:

> the current mortality tables are almost 70 years old. Tables now are based on the assumption that disabled vets die at an average age of 58, which is no longer true given today's record. As life expectancy has significantly improved over the past 60 years, commercial insurance companies have used up-to-date mortality tables. The newest table in general used by the insurance industry has premium rates roughly 50 percent lower than S-DVI rates.[54]

Because life expectancy has improved since the adoption of the S-DVI program, premiums based on the higher mortality rates of 1941 no longer fulfill congressional intent to provide life insurance to service-connected disabled veterans at standard rates. To address these concerns, it has been recommended that legislation be introduced to lower S-DVI premiums by basing them on the 2001 CSO Mortality Table (the table currently used by the National Association of Insurance Commissioners).

Some S-DVI policyholders are eligible for premium waivers at no extra cost. To be eligible for a premium waiver, an insured person must have a total disability that lasts six months or longer and that starts before the age of 65. Even if the total disability started before the effective date of the policy, a waiver can still be obtained as long as the total disability is service-connected.

Eligibility Requirements for Supplemental S-DVI ("Supplemental RH")

The Veterans' Benefits Act of 1992 (P.L. 102-568) made supplemental coverage accessible to S-DVI policyholders. Veterans who are totally disabled may apply for a waiver of premiums and additional supplemental coverage of up to $20,000. The Veterans' Benefits Act of 2010 (P.L. 111-275) increased the maximum coverage amount to $30,000 effective October 1, 2011. However, premiums cannot be waived on the additional supplemental coverage. To be eligible for Supplemental RH, policyholders must meet the following eligibility requirements:

- They are eligible for a waiver of premiums on their basic S-DVI policy due to total disability;[55]
- They apply for this coverage within one year from notice of the grant of the waiver; and
- They are under the age of 65.[56]

In the 17-year period from December 1992 to September 2009, VA approved 36,200 applications for Supplemental RH.[57]

Gratuitous S-DVI ("ARH")

In 1959, Congress passed legislation to protect veterans who became incompetent due to a service-connected disability while eligible to apply for S-DVI, but who died before filing an application. This program is known as Gratuitous S-DVI (or ARH). Gratuitous S-DVI differs from S-DVI because it is

- issued posthumously;[58]
- payable to a preferred class of a veteran's relatives; and
- payable in a lump sum.[59]

Eligibility Requirements for Gratuitous S-DVI

Gratuitous S-DVI is granted posthumously to veterans who

- met the basic eligibility requirements for S-DVI;
- did not apply for S-DVI because of continued mental incompetence due to a service-connected disability; and
- died before a guardian was appointed or within two years of such appointment.[60]

Applicants must submit their applications for Gratuitous S-DVI payment within two years from the date of the veteran's death. But if the person making the claim is mentally or legally incompetent when the right to apply for the benefit expires, he or she may apply within one year after his or her incompetency ends.

Gratuitous S-DVI lets veterans' families obtain lump-sum payments of $10,000 after the veterans' deaths as long as the previously mentioned eligibility requirements have been met. Gratuitous S-DVI is only payable as a lump sum and may not be paid as an annuity.

Payment of Gratuitous S-DVI is made to the following family members in the order listed below:

1. widow or widower of the insured, if living; if not
2. insured's child or children, if living, in equal shares; if not
3. insured's parents, if living, in equal shares.[61]

Management and Administration

In 1919, the VA began oversight of all servicemember life insurance programs. The VA issued United States Government Life Insurance to WWI servicemembers (1919-1951), National Service Life Insurance for WWII servicemembers (1940-1951), Veterans' Special Life Insurance for Korean War servicemembers (1951-1956), and Veterans' Reopened Life Insurance for disabled WWII and Korean War servicemembers (1965-1966). All of these life insurance programs are currently closed to new issues. The only three VA life insurance programs that provide benefits to the families of servicemembers and veterans, and that are still allowing new issues of life insurance, are S-DVI, SGLI, and VGLI. Congress passed the Insurance Act of 1951 (P.L. 82-23) and established the S-DVI program. S-DVI was created to meet the insurance needs of certain veterans with service-connected disabilities, many of whom would not be eligible for private life insurance due to their service-connected disabilities. Following S-DVI, in 1965, with the authorization of Congress (as part of establishing SGLI), the VA Administrator purchased group life insurance and selected the Prudential Insurance Company of America to cover its policies. In 1974, VGLI became available to former servicemembers (P.L. 93-289). VGLI provides for the conversion of SGLI after separation from active duty.

In 1965, the Advisory Council on Servicemembers' Group Life Insurance was established.[62] Initially, the Advisory Council is responsible for reviewing the SGLI programs and advising the Secretary of Veterans Affairs on policy matters concerning SGLI. However, in 1974, the Advisory Council became responsible for reviewing the VGLI program as well. The Advisory Council consists of the following six members according to current law:

- Secretary of the Treasury as chairperson;
- Secretary of Defense;
- Secretary of Commerce;
- Secretary of Health and Human Services;
- Secretary of Homeland Security; and
- Director of the Office of Management and Budget.

The VA Regional Office and Insurance Center (VAROIC) in Philadelphia, PA, supervises the SGLI and VGLI programs. However, the OSGLI in Roseland, NJ, a division of Prudential, administers the day-to-day operations of SGLI and VGLI.

How Policy Proceeds are Paid Out: Alliance Account

SGLI and VGLI policyholders may choose to have their benefits paid via Alliance Accounts. The Alliance Account is an interest-bearing retained asset account administered through the Prudential Insurance Company of America that is similar to a checking account. Like a checking account, proceeds are deposited in the beneficiary's name and he or she is given a draft book, which the beneficiary may use to write drafts for any amount up to the full amount of the proceeds. However, unlike checks, drafts may not be used to make purchases at the point of sale. Instead, the beneficiary must write the draft and deposit it into his or her checking account where the money will be transferred from the beneficiary's Alliance Account.[63] According to the VA, more than 60,000 Alliance Accounts have been opened and successfully managed since 1999.[64]

Servicemembers may have their SGLI and VGLI proceeds paid either as a lump sum or over a period of 36 months. The pay-out decision can only be made by the member at the time that he or she fills out the Servicemembers' Group Life Insurance Election and Certificate (SGLI 8286) Form. Since 1999, if the member chose to have his or her benefits paid as a lump sum without specifying that the payment be made via a single check, beneficiaries would have automatically received payments via Alliance Accounts. However, in light of recent media coverage condemning this practice as a violation of contractual agreements, Prudential now plans to send beneficiaries of VA life-insurance policies a check when they ask for a lump-sum benefit payment rather than keeping the money in an Alliance Account and mailing a checkbook, unless the policyholder specifically requests an Alliance Account.

Alliance Accounts are not offered under the S-DVI program, which is administered entirely by the VA. S-DVI beneficiaries may receive a lump-sum check payment or monthly payments, as predetermined by the veteran at the time that he or she fills out the application.

Accelerated Benefit Option

SGLI or VGLI policyholders may have access to the death benefits of their policies before they die if they exercise the Accelerated Benefit Option (ABO). This is a one-time benefit, available only if the policyholder is deemed terminally ill. If exercised, the ABO allows the member to receive a lump-sum payment of the insurance subject to the following:

- Terminally ill policyholders will have access of up to 50% of the face amount of their coverage during their lifetime.
- This money will be available in increments of $5,000.
- The insured must have a medical prognosis of life expectancy of nine months or less.[65]

The S-DVI program does not have an ABO.

Financial Counseling

Since October 1, 1999, the Free Financial Counseling Service (FFCS) has been available to VA insurance program beneficiaries. FFCS is a benefit that provides personalized objective financial counseling to SGLI, VGLI, and TSGLI[66] beneficiaries at no additional charge. VA reports that the average participation rate for FFCS is approximately 9%.

FFCS is provided by ComPsych, an outside vendor that offers financial counseling to beneficiaries under the product name FinancialPoint. Prudential contracts with FinancialPoint, and all counseling expenses concerning SGLI beneficiaries are charged to the SGLI program. According to the VA, expense charges for Policy Year 2009 were appro-ximately $249,000.[67]

Financial counseling is available to beneficiaries under FinancialPoint as long as they have an Alliance Account. Beneficiaries may contact financial advisors to answer financial questions 24 hours a day, seven days a week, by calling FinancialPoint's toll free number or by e-mail.[68] According to ComPsych, FinancialPoint advisors do not sell any products to beneficiaries and receive no commissions for their services. Beneficiaries may request targeted assistance; for instance, help with estate planning or saving for retirement. Beneficiaries may also request a comprehensive personalized financial plan by submitting a detailed financial questionnaire or having a face-to-face meeting with an advisor.

POLICY ISSUES

Lack of Transparency for SGLI and VGLI Policyholders

The VA agreed in September 2009 to allow Prudential Financial to provide payments of lump-sum benefits through Prudential's Alliance Accounts (a retained asset account) unless the beneficiary elects a single check. These funds were withheld in Alliance Accounts and invested by Prudential Financial for a profit. Recent media coverage has condemned this practice as deceptive and a violation of contractual agreements established by the VA. Another concern about Alliance Accounts is that they are not insured by the Federal Deposit Insurance Corporation (FDIC). This may put beneficiaries at risk of losing their benefits in the event that Prudential's financial investments fail. Legislation has been introduced in the 111th Congress concerning this issue. H.R. 5993 and S. 3718 were introduced to ensure that beneficiaries of Servicemembers' Group Life Insurance receive financial counseling and disclosure information regarding life insurance payments, and for other purposes. H.R. 5993 was reported on September 28, 2010 (H.Rept. 111-628).

Because of the recent media coverage, the VA has been proactive, taking action to revamp its claims materials, to create more transparency for SGLI and VGLI beneficiaries, and to require payments of lump-sum benefits through a single check unless the beneficiary elects to use an Alliance Account.[69] To improve its existing claim forms, the VA plans to add new documents that give beneficiaries the opportunity to choose their payment option, including a lump-sum check, a lump-sum Alliance Account, or 36 monthly installments.[70] The VA also plans to continue to provide a full explanation of its terms up front and begin highlighting that the Alliance Accounts are not covered by the FDIC.

> Prudential has agreed to implement these adjustments, and the department plans to continue to carefully monitor this program to ensure that Servicemembers' and Veterans' beneficiaries are well-protected.[71]

Other actions that the VA is planning to take include

- modifying all SGLI and VGLI related information, including frequently asked questions, website information, and handbooks in order to clearly and completely explain all aspects of the Alliance Account and all options available to the beneficiary;
- establishing requirements for Prudential to conduct a follow-up contact with beneficiaries whose accounts remain open after six months to confirm the beneficiary understands the terms of the account;
- clearly designating the source of correspondence by removing the SGLI seal from all checks, forms, and correspondence and replacing it to show that it is from Prudential, with the subtitle of "Office of Servicemembers' Group Life Insurance";
- identifying additional opportunities to encourage beneficiaries to use the free financial counseling service; and
- improving support to Casualty Assistant Officers and Transition Assistance Program (TAP) Personnel by helping to prepare additional training materials and instruction in coordination with the DOD.

Coverage Limit for S-DVI

Currently, S-DVI policies are issued for a maximum face value of $10,000. This amount has not been increased in almost six decades. The $10,000 maximum coverage was part of the S-DVI program at its inception in 1951.[72] By comparison, $10,000 in 1951 would be worth nearly $84,000 in 2010 after adjusting for inflation. Also, policyholders are denied the opportunity to buy additional coverage under the program.[73]

As of June 24, 2009, less than 4% of veterans who were eligible to participate in the program were insured under S-DVI.[74] According to a recent congressionally mandated study, the lowest area of veteran satisfaction was "the maximum amount of S-DVI insurance coverage that veterans were authorized to purchase."[75] Some critics say the program falls far short of delivering the protection it was originally designed to provide. For example, Brian E. Lawrence, assistant national legislative director of the Disabled American Veterans, said

> Government life insurance programs have limited basic coverage to $10,000 since their inception under the War Risk Insurance Act in 1917. Then, they were an excellent benefit. More than 93 percent of military members adopted the maximum coverage of $10,000 because they knew that in the event of their death, their family members would have the financial resources available to pay for the cost of a home and also to cover the cost of living for a considerable amount of time. For example, Sears, Roebuck and Co. sold prefabricated houses in the early 1900's. Its 1920 catalogue featured 80 models, ranging in price from $4,900 to $6,000. Obviously, $10,000 went much further in 1917 than it does in 2003.[76]

According to the VA, 46% of the veterans enrolled in the S-DVI program are considered totally disabled and are eligible for a premium waiver for their basic coverage.[77] Of those who are eligible, only 27% currently have a Supplemental S-DVI policy, which provides an additional $20,000 in coverage.[78] This means that about 12% of all S-DVI policyholders have

$30,000 in total coverage, while the remaining 88% of participants have $10,000 in total coverage. Put in perspective, the VGLI program offers maximum coverage of $400,000. Legislation has been introduced in the 111th Congress to change the amounts of coverage for which S-DVI participants are eligible. S. 728, H.R. 2713, and H.R. 1037 as amended by the Senate are examples of legislation that primarily focus on increasing the amount of coverage available to disabled veterans and replacing the use of the outdated (1941) mortality table when determining the premium amounts for veterans.

Additionally, because coverage for S-DVI is not wholly funded by the premiums paid by policyholders, Congress appropriates funds to subsidize the program. These appropriations are necessary to support veterans who are waived from paying premiums because they are totally disabled from service-connected disabilities. Therefore, if the amount of coverage available to veterans were to increase the appropriation allocated for the S-DVI program would also have to increase in order to avoid facing a short fall. In FY2010, Congress appropriated approximately $40.1 million for veterans covered under the S-DVI program.

End Notes

[1] A retained asset account is a bank account established in the beneficiary's name that provides the insurer with a means to retain (withhold) assets for investment purposes. Beneficiaries receive a personalized draft book which they can use to withdraw funds from the retained asset account for up to the full amount of benefits available.

[2] Department of Veterans Affairs, "VA Continues to Ensure and Protect Servicemembers', Survivors' Life Insurance Benefits," press release, September 14, 2010, http://www1.va.gov/opa/pressrel/pressrelease.cfm?id=1956.

[3] The term "servicemember" refers to a person on active duty, active duty for training, or inactive duty training in the uniformed services in a commissioned, warrant, or enlisted rank, or grade, or as a cadet or midshipman of the United States Military Academy, United States Naval Academy, United States Air Force Academy, or the United States Coast Guard Academy.

[4] Department of Veterans Affairs, Regional Office and Insurance Center, *VA Life Insurance Programs for Veterans and Servicemembers,* Philadelphia, PA, January 2010, p. 31, http://www.insurance.va.gov/gli/glihandbook/glibooklet2010.pdf.

[5] Traumatic Injuries are discussed further in the text under the heading "SGLI Traumatic Injury Protection Program." Also, see 38 C.F.R. § 9.20 for more information on Traumatic Injuries.

[6] "Full-time" or "Part-time" coverage depends on level of active military service.

[7] Title 10 of the *U.S. Code* includes laws relating to the U.S. Armed Forces.

[8] Department of Veterans Affairs, *Servicemembers' and Veterans' Group Life Insurance Handbook,* H-29-98-1, Washington, DC, August 2009, p. 6, http://www.insurance.va.gov/sgliSite/handbook/handbook.pdf.

[9] Title 32 of the *U.S. Code* includes laws relating to the National Guard.

[10] Department of Veterans Affairs, *Servicemembers' and Veterans' Group Life Insurance Handbook,* H-29-98-1, Washington, DC, August 2009, pp. 6-7, http://www.insurance.va.gov/sgliSite/handbook/handbook.pdf.

[11] The most recent change to SGLI maximum coverage amount was made on September 1, 2005.

[12] This form can be found on the VA Website at https://www.insurance.va.gov/sgliSite/converting/FSGLI.htm.

[13] "Proof of good health" shall be submitted at the applicant's own expense (38 U.S.C. § 1977(g)).

[14] 38 U.S.C. § 1967(c).

[15] 38 U.S.C. § 1973.

[16] 38 U.S.C. § 1967, and § 1968.

[17] Department of Veterans Affairs, *Servicemembers' and Veterans' Group Life Insurance Handbook*, H-29-98-1, Washington, DC, August 2009, p. 8, http://www.insurance.va.gov/sgliSite/handbook/handbook.pdf.

[18] Department of Veterans Affairs, Regional Office and Insurance Center, *VA Life Insurance Programs for Veterans and Servicemembers,* Philadelphia, PA, January 2010, p. 33, http://www.insurance.va.gov/gli/glihandbook/glibooklet2010.pdf. Also, a list of participating companies is available at http://www.insurance.va.gov/sgliSite/forms/ sgl133ed07-10.pdf.

[19] 38 U.S.C. § 1967-1968.

[20] 38 U.S.C. § 1970(a).

[21] 38 U.S.C. § 1967(f). Also 38 C.F.R. § 9.40

[22] The most recent change to SGLI premium rates was made on July 1, 2008.

[23] Department of Veterans Affairs, Regional Office and Insurance Center, *VA Life Insurance Programs for Veterans and Servicemembers,* Philadelphia, PA, January 2010, p. 31, http://www.insurance.va.gov/gli/glihandbook/glibooklet2010.pdf.

[24] The term "extra hazards" refers to the amount of additional monies required to pay death claims that exceed those that would be incurred under normal peacetime conditions.

[25] Department of Veterans Affairs, Regional Office and Insurance Center, *Servicemembers' and Veterans' Group Life Insurance Programs: Forty-Fourth Annual Report,* Philadelphia, PA, June 2009, pp. 6-7, https://www.insurance.va.gov/sgliSite/miscellaneous/SGLI-Ann-Report-2009.pdf.

[26] 38 U.S.C. § 1969.

[27] This form can be found on the VA Website at https://www.insurance.va.gov/sgliSite/converting/FSGLI.htm.

[28] Department of Veterans Affairs, *Servicemembers' and Veterans' Group Life Insurance Handbook,* H-29-98-1 Washington, DC, August 2009, p. 36, http://www.insurance.va.gov/sgliSite/handbook/handbook.pdf.

[29] Department of Veterans Affairs, *Servicemembers' and Veterans' Group Life Insurance Handbook,* H-29-98-1 Washington, DC, August 2009, pp. 34-37, http://www.insurance.va.gov/sgliSite/handbook/handbook.pdf.

[30] Department of Veterans Affairs, Regional Office and Insurance Center, *Servicemembers' and Veterans' Group Life Insurance Programs: Forty-Fourth Annual Report,* Philadelphia, PA, June 2009, p. 4, https://www.insurance.va.gov/ sgliSite/miscellaneous/SGLI-Ann-Report-2009.pdf.

[31] Ibid., p. 38.

[32] Ibid., pp. 36-38.

[33] Department of Veterans Affairs, Regional Office and Insurance Center, *VA Life Insurance Programs for Veterans and Servicemembers,* Philadelphia, PA, January 2010, pp. 34-35, http://www.insurance.va.gov/gli/glihandbook/ glibooklet2010.pdf. Also 38 U.S.C. § 9.20.

[34] Ibid., p. 34.

[35] Department of Veterans Affairs, *Servicemembers' and Veterans' Group Life Insurance Handbook,* H-29-98-1 Washington, DC, August 2009, pp. 42-43, http://www.insurance.va.gov/sgliSite/handbook/handbook.pdf.

[36] The phrase "inability to perform two activities of daily living" means the inability to independently perform two or more of the following six functions: Bathing, continence, dressing, eating, toileting, or transferring.

[37] Department of Veterans Affairs, Regional Office and Insurance Center, *VA Life Insurance Programs for Veterans and Servicemembers,* Philadelphia, PA, January 2010, p. 35, http://www.insurance.va.gov/gli/glihandbook/glibooklet2010.pdf.

[38] Ibid.

[39] Ibid., p. 34.

[40] TSGLI is not an optional program.

[41] A list of participating companies is available at http://www.insurance.va.gov/sgliSite/forms/sgl133ed07-10.pdf.

[42] Members who join the Ready Reserves/National Guard after release from active duty are eligible to continue their SGLI coverage for as long as they remain in the Ready Reserves/National Guard. They are also eligible to convert their active duty SGLI coverage to VGLI coverage.

[43] Department of Veterans Affairs, *Servicemembers and Veterans Group Life Insurance Handbook*, H-29-98-1, Washington, DC, August 2009, p. 47, http://www.insurance.va.gov/sgliSite/handbook/handbook.pdf.

[44] Any impairment of mind or body which continuously renders it impossible for the insured to follow any substantially gainful occupation; the permanent loss or loss of use of both feet, or both hands, or both eyes, or one foot and one hand, or one hand and one eye; the total loss of hearing in both ears; or the organic loss of speech. Veterans having any of the before mentioned disabilities are considered totally disabled regardless of employment. Members having other disabilities are considered totally disabled only when the disability would prevent the member from engaging in substantially gainful employment.

[45] The two-year period for conversion from SGLI to VGLI for disabled servicemembers was made permanent by the Veterans' Benefits Act of 2010 (P.L. 111-275) and is effective for separations from service after June 14, 2005.

[46] The first five-year period begins on the one-year anniversary of the date the member becomes insured under VGLI.

[47] Department of Veterans Affairs, Regional Office and Insurance Center, *VA Life Insurance Programs for Veterans and Servicemembers*, Philadelphia, PA, January 2010, p. 42, https://www.insurance.va.gov/gli/glihandbook/glibooklet2010.pdf.

[48] A list of participating companies is available at http://www.insurance.va.gov/sgliSite/forms/sgl133ed07-10.pdf.

[49] 38 U.S.C. § 101.

[50] Barry A. Searle, "VA Service-Disabled Veterans Insurance," *American Legion Bulletin*, Washington, DC, December 3, 2009, p. 1, http://www.missourilegion.org/30-09%20sdvi%20bulletin%20dec%2009%20(2).pdf.

[51] If the veteran has been released for bad conduct discharge awarded at Special Court-Martial he or she may be eligible if the administering agency determines that, for its purposes, the discharge was not under dishonorable conditions.

[52] Service-connected disabilities are evaluated according to the VA Schedule for Rating Disabilities in Title 38, *Code of Federal Regulations*, Part 4.

[53] Department of Veterans Affairs, Regional Office and Insurance Center, *VA Life Insurance Programs for Veterans and Servicemembers*, Philadelphia, PA, January 2010, p. 24, http://www.insurance.va.gov/gli/glihandbook/glibooklet2010.pdf.

[54] U.S. Congress, House Committee on Veterans' Affairs, Subcommittee on Disability Assistance and Memorial Affairs, *Legislative Hearing on H.R. 2379, H.R. 2713, H.R. 2774, and H.R. 2968*, 111th Cong., 1st sess., June 24, 2009, Serial No. 111-31 (Washington: GPO, 2010), p. 2.

[55] Total disability means the veteran is unable to work on his or her own at any occupation for which he or she is suited by training, education, or experience.

[56] Department of Veterans Affairs, Regional Office and Insurance Center, *VA Life Insurance Programs for Veterans and Servicemembers*, Philadelphia, PA, January 2010, p. 23, http://www.insurance.va.gov/gli/glihandbook/glibooklet2010.pdf.

[57] Ibid.

[58] After death.

[59] Department of Veterans Affairs, Regional Office and Insurance Center, *VA Life Insurance Programs for Veterans and Servicemembers*, Philadelphia, PA, January 2010, p. 24, http://www.insurance.va.gov/gli/glihandbook/glibooklet2010.pdf.

[60] Ibid., p. 75.

[61] Ibid.

[62] 38 U.S.C. § 1974.

[63] Beneficiaries cannot deposit additional funds into an Alliance Account.

[64] U.S. Department of Veterans Affairs, *Fact Sheet: Servicemembers' Group Life Insurance (SGLI) and Veterans Group Life Insurance (VGLI) Programs and the Alliance Accounts Operated by the Prudential Insurance Company of America*, August 4, 2010, p. 2.

[65] Department of Veterans Affairs, Regional Office and Insurance Center, *VA Life Insurance Programs for Veterans and Servicemembers*, Philadelphia, PA, January 2010, p. 33, https://www.insurance.va.gov/gli/glihandbook/glibooklet2010.pdf.

[66] The TSGLI program is administered under SGLI program and provides short-term financial assistance to servicemembers who suffer from traumatic injuries.

[67] July 1, 2008 through June 30, 2009.

[68] 1-888-243-7351 (SGLI or VGLI) or 1-800-428-3416 (TSGLI) or fcs@FinancialPoint.com.

[69] Department of Veterans Affairs, "VA Continues to Ensure and Protect Servicemembers', Survivors' Life Insurance Benefits," press release, September 14, 2010, http://www1.va.gov/opa/pressrel/pressrelease.cfm?id=1956.

[70] Under the existing setup, the option to request a check in the mail is not on the claims form.

[71] Statement by Veterans Affairs Chief of Staff John R. Gingrich, Department of Veterans Affairs, "VA Continues to Ensure and Protect Servicemembers', Survivors' Life Insurance Benefits," press release, September 14, 2010, http://www1.va.gov/opa/pressrel/pressrelease.cfm?id=1956.

[72] U.S. Congress, House Committee on Veterans' Affairs, Subcommittee on Disability Assistance and Memorial Affairs, *Legislative Hearing on H.R. 2379, H.R. 2713, H.R. 2774, and H.R. 2968*, 111th Cong., 1st sess., June 24, 2009, Serial No. 111-31 (Washington: GPO, 2010), p. 5.

[73] Ibid., p. 2.

[74] U.S. Congress, House Committee on Veterans Affairs, Subcommittee on Disability Assistance and Memorial Affairs, *Legislative Hearing on H.R. 2379, H.R. 2713, H.R. 2774, and H.R. 2968*, 111th Cong., 1st sess., June 24, 2009, Serial No. 111-31 (Washington: GPO, 2009), p. 2.

[75] Department of Veterans Affairs, *Program Evaluation of Benefits for Survivors of Veterans with Service-Connected Disabilities.*

[76] U.S. Congress, House Committee on Veterans' Affairs, Subcommittee on Benefits, *Oversight Hearing on the Department of Veterans Affairs Life Insurance Program*, 108th Cong., 1st sess., September 25, 2003, Serial No. 108-23 (Washington: GPO, 2004), p. 10, http://veterans.house.gov/hearings/schedule108/sep03/9-25-03/9-25b-03.pdf.

[77] Department of Veterans Affairs, *VA Life Insurance Programs for Veterans and Servicemen*, Philadelphia, PA, January 2010, p. 26, http://www.insurance.va.gov/gli/glihandbook/glibooklet2010.pdf.

[78] U.S. Congress, Senate Committee on Veterans' Affairs, *Veterans Benefits Enhancement Act of 2009,* report to accompany S. 728, 111th Cong., 1st sess., September 2, 2009, S.Rept. 111-71 (Washington: GPO, 2009), p. 3.

In: Veterans Benefits
Editors: George B. Meyers and Alice M. Glaskin
ISBN: 978-1-61209-581-3

Chapter 8

VETERANS BENEFITS: FEDERAL EMPLOYMENT ASSISTANCE

Christine Scott

SUMMARY

There are federal employment and training programs and policies specifically targeted to help veterans seeking employment in the civilian economy. Transition assistance programs are operated by the Department of Defense (DOD), the Department of Veterans Affairs (VA), and the Department of Labor (DOL) to assist servicemembers as they prepare to leave the military. DOL operates grant programs to states to provide outreach and assistance to veterans in finding civilian employment. In addition, the federal government has policies (including veterans preference) that assist veterans in obtaining jobs with the federal government and federal contractors. This chapter provides a brief overview of these federal programs and policies.

Veterans may participate in the general employment and training programs open to Veveryone seeking jobs, or in certain programs targeted specifically to veterans.[1] In addition, the federal government has a policy of assisting veterans in employment through the use of preferences in federal employment, and requirements for affirmative action in the hiring of veterans by federal contractors. This chapter will provide an overview of these federal employment and training programs targeted to veterans, and federal policies to assist veterans in obtaining federal employment.[2]

CASH ASSISTANCE

Part of the Servicemen's Readjustment Act of 1944 (The GI Bill, P.L. 78-346) provided a cash allowance for returning unemployed veterans. This was provided because, at the time, veterans were not eligible for unemployment compensation. However, because of a combination of factors, including the strong economic growth shortly after World War II and the GI Bill's education and training benefits, few veterans took advantage of the cash assistance program.

WHEN IS A DISCHARGED SERVICEMEMBER CLASSIFIED AS A "VETERAN" FOR THE PURPOSES OF VA BENEFITS?

Not all discharged servicemembers are considered "veterans" for the purposes of the Department of Veterans Affairs (VA) benefits and programs. In order to be eligible for most VA benefits, it is necessary for the discharged servicemember to be classified as a "veteran," or in some circumstances, the survivor of a veteran.

Federal statutes define "veteran" as a "person who served in the active military, naval, or air service, and who was discharged or released therefrom under conditions other than dishonorable." [38 U.S.C. § 101(2); 38 C.F.R. § 3.1(d)]. The VA largely bases its determination of veteran status upon military department service records. In addition to the member's service records, other factors impact his/her classification as a "veteran" and may impact future benefits. These factors include

- *Discharge criteria:* (38 U.S.C. § 101(2); 38 C.F.R. § 3.1(d)).
- *Active military, naval or air service:* (38 U.S.C. § 101(2); 38 C.F.R. § 3.1(d)).
- *Whether the service was during "time of war:"* (38 U.S.C. § 101(6)-(11); 38 C.F.R. § 3.2).
- *Length of duty requirement:* (38 U.S.C. § 101(6)-(11); 38 C.F.R. § 3.2).

After it has been proved that the discharged servicemember meets these criteria, he/she is considered to be a "veteran" and may be eligible for certain benefits relating to health care, education, and other services which are provided by the VA.

(Information provided by Douglas Reid Weimer, Legislative Attorney, American Law Division, CRS.)

There is currently no system to provide a cash allowance to veterans seeking civilian employment although veterans are eligible for unemployment compensation, which provides partial replacement of lost cash wages.[3]

EMPLOYMENT ASSISTANCE

The federal government operates programs to assist veterans seeking civilian employment and provides preferences in federal employment for veterans. Outlined below are the major federal programs and policies to assist veterans seeking civilian jobs.

Transition Assistance Programs

The Department of Labor (DOL), in cooperation with the Department of Defense (DOD) and the VA, operates the Transition Assistance Program (TAP) and Disabled Transition Assistance Program (DTAP). Both programs are designed to provide information on employment and training for servicemembers within 180 days of separation from military service, or retirement.[4]

TAP is a three-day workshop conducted at military installations that includes sessions on how to look for jobs, current market conditions (both labor market and occupation-specific information is provided), preparation of job search materials (including resumes), and interview techniques. DTAP adds additional hours to the three-day program focused on the special needs of disabled servicemembers.

In addition to the employment assistance sessions, information is provided on veterans benefits administered by the VA.

Veterans State Grants Program

The DOL Veterans' Employment and Training Service (VETS) offers assistance to veterans seeking jobs through the Jobs for Veterans State Grants (JVSG) Program. Under the program, grants are used to fund Disabled Veterans' Outreach Program (DVOP) specialists and Local Veterans' Employment Representatives (LVER).[5] These are state positions, funded by the federal government, that provide outreach and assistance to veterans seeking employment.

DVOP staff in a state are involved in outreach efforts to disabled veterans with greater barriers to employment, who therefore need more intensive services for employment or training. LVER staff help veterans find employment and are involved in outreach to the business community to encourage the hiring of veterans (including disabled veterans).

Veterans' Workforce Investment Program

The VETS office also operates the Veterans' Workforce Investment Program (VWIP), a grant program authorized under the Workforce Investment Act (WIA, P.L. 105-220).[6] Grants may be made to fund programs operated by eligible state and local workforce investment boards, state or local agencies, or private non-profit organizations. The grants are intended to help reintegrate veterans into the civilian labor force; develop service delivery systems that address the needs of veterans entering the civilian workforce; enhance workforce investment activities related to veterans; and perform outreach or public information activities to promote employment of veterans.

In addition to the JVSG Program and the VWIP program, the VETS office in DOL also

- conducts the *HireVetsFirst* campaign to encourage employers to hire veterans;
- provides grants under the Homeless Veterans Reintegration Program;[7] and

- provides information to veterans and employers on re-employment rights under the Uniformed Services Employment and Reemployment Rights Act of 1994 (USERRA, P.L. 103-353).

All VETS activities are required partners in the One-Stop Career Center system established by WIA.[8]

Any workforce development, job training, or placement program funded in part by DOL must provide a priority in services for veterans and eligible spouses. In general, persons covered under the priority of service (veterans and spouses) receive access to services and resources before non-covered persons.[9]

America's Heroes at Work

In January 2009, the DOL began a new pilot program, America's Heroes at Work, for veterans with traumatic brain injury (TBI) or post-traumatic stress disorder (PTSD). Under the pilot program, DOL will study, validate, and disseminate best practices related to helping employees with TBI or PTSD succeed on the job. The website for the program provides information and fact sheets for employers and veterans on topics related to TBI and PTSD, including how employers can make accommodations in their workplace for impacted employees.[10]

Federal Employment Preferences

The federal government has four policies that provide a preference to veterans: (1) a system of point preference for hiring; (2) special appointment (hiring) authority; (3) affirmative action requirements for federal agencies; and (4) affirmative action requirements for contractors and subcontractors.[11]

Point Preference

Veterans are given a federal preference in hiring to prevent an individual from being penalized for having spent time in military federal service. A five-point preference is given to veterans with an honorable or general discharge who served on active duty (not active duty for training):

- during any war;
- during the period April 28, 1952, through July 1, 1955;
- for more than 180 consecutive days, any part of which occurred after January 31, 1955, and before October 15, 1976;
- during the Gulf War period beginning August 2, 1990, and ending January 2, 1992;
- for more than 180 consecutive days, any part of which occurred during the period beginning September 11, 2001, and ending on the date prescribed by presidential proclamation or by law as the last day of Operation Iraqi Freedom; or

- in a campaign or expedition for which a campaign medal has been authorized, such as El Salvador, Lebanon, Grenada, Panama, Southwest Asia, Somalia, and Haiti.

To qualify for a five-point preference, medal holders and Gulf War veterans who originally enlisted after September 7, 1980, or entered on active duty on or after October 14, 1982, without having previously completed 24 months of continuous active duty, must have served continuously for 24 months or the full period called or ordered to active duty. As of October 1, 1980, military retirees at or above the rank of major or equivalent are not entitled to preference unless they qualify as disabled veterans.

A ten-point preference is given to

- honorably separated veterans who qualify as disabled veterans because they have served on active duty in the Armed Forces at any time and have a present service-connected disability or are receiving compensation, disability retirement benefits, or pension from the military or the Department of Veterans Affairs;
- honorably separated veterans who are Purple Heart recipients;
- the spouse of a veteran unable to work because of a service-connected disability;
- the unmarried widow of certain deceased veterans; and
- certain mothers of veterans who died in service or who are permanently and totally disabled.[12]

Special Appointment (Hiring) Authority

There are three special appointment authorities available to federal government agencies related to veterans: (1) Veterans Recruitment Appointment (VRA); (2) Veterans Employment Opportunity Acts (VEOA); and (3) 30% or More Disabled Veteran (30%).

Veterans Recruitment Appointment (VRA)

The use of a VRA allows agencies to appoint an eligible veteran without competition. The VRA is an excepted appointment to a position that is otherwise in the competitive service. After two years of satisfactory service, the veteran may be converted to a career-conditional appointment in the competitive service.[13]

Once in federal employment, VRAs are treated like any other competitive service employee and may be promoted, reassigned, or transferred. VRA appointees with less than 15 years of education must complete a training program established by the agency. Veterans eligible for a VRA appointment are

- disabled veterans;
- veterans who served on active duty in the Armed Forces during a war, or in a campaign or expedition for which a campaign badge has been authorized;
- veterans who, while serving on active duty in the Armed Forces, participated in a United States military operation for which an Armed Forces Service Medal was awarded; or
- recently separated veterans.

In addition to meeting the criteria above, veterans must have been separated under honorable conditions (i.e., the individual must have received either an honorable or general discharge).

Veterans Employment Opportunity Act (VEOA)

Federal agencies can recruit outside their own workforce, to all competitive service employees, in filling permanent competitive service openings. Veterans are eligible to apply for this type of open position even if not a current competitive service employee if the veteran is a preference eligible or has completed three or more years of active service. The federal government agency can then appoint the veteran using the VEOA appointment authority.

30% or More Disabled Veteran

The 30% or more disabled veteran authority allows a federal government agency to noncompetitively appoint any veteran with a 30% or more service-connected disability to a permanent, temporary (one year or less), or term (one to four years) positions in the competitive service. For permanent appointments, the veteran is placed in a time limited (60 days maximum) appointment and then converted to permanent at management's discretion.

Affirmative Action: Federal Agencies

Federal agencies must have a separate affirmative action program for disabled veterans as part of agency efforts to hire, place, and advance persons with disabilities under the Rehabilitation Act of 1973 (P.L. 93-112).[14] Agencies are required to

- provide placement consideration under special noncompetitive hiring authorities for VRAs and veterans with a disability rating of 30% or more;
- ensure that all veterans are considered for employment and advancement under merit system rules; and
- establish an affirmative action plan for the hiring, placement, and advancement of disabled veterans.

Affirmative Action: Contractors and Subcontractors

Contractors and subcontractors with federal contracts in excess of $100,000 must report to the DOL on efforts to hire veterans in specific categories: disabled veterans, other protected veterans, Armed Forces service medal veterans, and recently separated veterans. Contractors and subcontractors are required to post job openings through state job services or one stop offices, and may post job openings on the federal online service (America's Job Bank).[15]

Veterans Hiring Initiative

On November 9, 2009, President Obama issued Executive Order 13518, which established a Veterans Hiring Initiative and established a Council on Veterans Employment co-chaired by the Secretaries of DOL and VA. As part of the initiative, the Office of Personnel Management (OPM) established a new website—http://www.fedshirevets.gov—to provide information for veterans on federal government employment. One of the features of the website is an agency directory providing for each agency, the name, email address, and telephone number of the individual within each agency responsible for promoting veterans' employment within the agency.

Other Federal Assistance

The Department of Defense Appropriations Act, 2003 (P.L. 107-248) authorized the DOD to transfer funds to the Center for Military Recruitment, Assessment, and Veterans Employment. The center is a 501(c)(6) organization supported by construction employers and building and trade organizations within the AFL-CIO to help veterans find employment in the construction industry, through operation of the "Helmets to Hardhats" program.[16] The transfer of funds has been done each year since FY2003, with the FY2010 transfer being $3.0 million as provided by the Department of Defense Appropriations Act (P.L. 111-118).

The Department of Education transfers funds to the DOD to provide funding for participants in the "Troops 2 Teachers" Program. The program can provide a stipend of up to $5,000 for eligible military personnel to obtain certification as an elementary, secondary, or vocational/technical teacher. Instead of the stipend for certification, the program may pay a bonus of up to $10,000 to participants who teach in a high-poverty school. For FY2010, the funding for the program is $14 million.

End Notes

[1] This chapter does not address federal employment and training programs open to everyone seeking jobs.

[2] This paper does not provide information on VA education benefits for veterans. For more information on education benefits for veterans see CRS Report R40723, *Educational Assistance Programs Administered by the U.S. Department of Veterans Affairs*, by Cassandria Dortch.

[3] For more information on unemployment compensation for veterans, see CRS Report RS22440, *Unemployment Compensation (Insurance) and Military Service*, by Julie M. Whittaker.

[4] For more information on TAP and DTAP programs, see the Department of Labor's TAP Fact Sheet at http://www.dol.gov/vets/programs/tap/tap_fs.htm.

[5] For information on LVER and DVOP grants, see the DOL guide to grants at http://www.dol.gov/vets/grants/Final_VETS_Guide-linked.pdf.

[6] Ibid. (For information on VWIP grants).

[7] For more information on the program, please see CRS Report RL34024, *Veterans and Homelessness*, by Libby Perl.

[8] Local one-stop service centers can be found online at http://www.servicelocator.org/.

[9] Regulations on the priority of service can be found at http://www.dol.gov/vets/E8-30166.pdf.

[10] The website for the program is http://www.americasheroesatwork.gov/.

[11] For federal employment purposes, a veteran is an individual who has active duty service, with minimum length of service requirements, for one of the time periods defined in Title 5, §2108. For more information on federal employment preferences for veterans, see the Office of Personnel Management's VetsInfo Guide at http://www.opm.gov/veterans/html/vetsinfo.asp.

[12] To receive the 10-point preference, the mother must be either: (1) married with a husband who is totally disabled; or (2) widowed, divorced, or separated at the time the 10-point preference is claimed (the mother loses the 10-point preference when she remarries).

[13] A veteran may be given a noncompetitive temporary or term appointment based on VRA eligibility. These appointments do not lead to career jobs.

[14] Each year the Office of Personnel Management (OPM) prepares a report with information on the accomplishments of affirmative action programs for disabled veterans. The OPM reports are available at http://www.opm.gov/veterans/ dvaap.asp.

[15] The federal online employment service can be found at http://www.usajobs.com/.

[16] For more Information, see the program website at http://www.helmetstohardhats.com/.

In: Veterans Benefits
Editors: George B. Meyers and Alice M. Glaskin
ISBN: 978-1-61209-581-3

Chapter 9

VETERANS' BENEFITS: THE VOCATIONAL REHABILITATION AND EMPLOYMENT PROGRAM

Christine Scott and Carol D. Davis

SUMMARY

The number of servicemembers, National Guard, and Reservists who separate from active duty with service-connected disabilities is expected to rise as a result of the engagement of the U.S. Armed Forces in Operation Iraqi Freedom and Operation Enduring Freedom. There is concern in Congress that these individuals receive the care and services that will enable them to transition successfully back to civilian life. These veterans must be able to rejoin their families and communities, become employed, and continue to enjoy the highest quality of life possible, given their disabilities.

Congress authorized the Department of Veterans Affairs (VA), through the Vocational Rehabilitation & Employment Service (VR&E), to provide the support disabled veterans need to successfully complete rehabilitation plans tailored to their individual needs. The VR&E has recently restructured its program in an effort to better accomplish the goal of enabling disabled veterans to gain appropriate employment or live independently. More specialists and counselors have been hired in regional VA offices, and the VR&E has instituted outreach efforts to encourage more veterans who might be eligible for these services to apply to participate in the program. The VR&E has also entered into cooperative agreements with other federal agencies, such as the Department of Labor and the Department of Education, and with private organizations to provide an integrated approach to addressing the employment needs of disabled servicemembers and veterans.

The VR&E administers four programs: (1) training and rehabilitation for veterans with service- connected disabilities; (2) vocational and educational counseling; (3) vocational training for Vietnam veterans' children with Spina Bifida; and (4) special restorative training. In addition, the Coming Home to Work Program of the VR&E Service is designed to facilitate the veteran's return to the work force with maximum speed. This chapter describes VR&E program services available to veterans with service-connected disabilities and to their families. It provides information about eligibility and entitlement, the application process, and resources available through other agencies. A brief history of the program is also provided.

Congress is concerned that servicemembers, National Guard, and Reservists involved in Operation Enduring Freedom and Operation Iraqi Freedom who are being discharged from military service with service-connected disabilities receive timely and effective vocational rehabilitation services. The Vocational Rehabilitation and Employment Program (VR&E), one of five major programs administered by the Veterans Benefits Administration (VBA) of the Department of Veterans Affairs (VA), addresses this concern.[1] The program's purpose is to counsel and rehabilitate veterans, with an emphasis on employment and independent living. The program provides comprehensive services and assistance to enable veterans with service-connected disabilities and employment handicaps[2] to achieve maximum independence in daily living, to become employable, and to obtain and maintain suitable employment. For severely disabled veterans, the goal is to help them achieve the highest quality of life possible with a future chance of employment, given medical and technological advances. The VR&E service delivery strategies differ from those of many other VBA programs as they require personal interaction with the veteran to deliver services and have the largest network of service delivery points of any VBA program.[3]

HISTORY

In 1918, Congress passed P.L. 65-178, the Vocational Rehabilitation Act, to provide for the retraining and placing in productive occupations of disabled persons who had served in the U.S. military and naval forces. The rehabilitation program was administered by the Federal Board for Vocational Education. On August 24, 1921, control of veterans' rehabilitation was transferred to the newly created Veterans' Bureau. In 1930, Congress created the Veterans Administration by combining three bureaus, the Veterans' Bureau, the Bureau of Pensions, and the National Homes for Disabled Volunteer Veterans.

In 1943, Congress passed P.L. 78-16, which provided that any eligible veteran may receive up to four years of training specifically directed to restoring employability. To be eligible for this training, the veteran must

- have been in the active military or naval service at any time after September 16, 1940, and during World War II;
- have been discharged under circumstances other than dishonorable;
- have a disability incurred in, or aggravated by, such service for which a pension is payable under the laws administered by the VA or would be but for the receipt of military retirement pay; and
- be in need of vocational rehabilitation to overcome the handicap caused by such service-connected disability.

Under this program, the VA provided services to 621,000 World War II disabled veterans.

Over the years, the scope of the VR&E program has been modified and expanded through legislation to better fulfill its mission. The program has undergone many name changes and has often been aligned with the education services of the VBA. In 1999, the program acquired its current name with the intention of placing more emphasis on employment services. Today, the VA handles the rehabilitation of disabled veterans through the VR&E program.

THE VR&E PROGRAM

In 2004, the Secretary of Veterans Affairs responded to continuing criticisms of the VR&E's operations from committees of Congress,[4] the Government Accountability Office (GAO), and others, by forming a task force to evaluate the program. The task force report[5] found little evidence that the program's efforts to obtain jobs for rehabilitated veterans had been as successful as intended by Congress. The task force felt that the VR&E staff was doing a good job for veterans; however, it also recognized the need for a more effective rehabilitation program to enable veterans to resume independent living and lead productive lives as soon as possible. According to the report, the foundation of the 21st century VR&E program should shift its focus to an individual's ability and away from an individual's disability. The task force report made 110 recommendations for the program's improvement. By the end of FY2007, over 89 of the 110 recommendations had been implemented.[6]

Before 1980, successful rehabilitation was defined as completion of a training program for suitable employment and not actual job placement. The task force identified this as an area that needed improvement. Under the current program, VR&E staff must make sure that a veteran understands that the primary goal of the VR&E program is employment and encourage and motivate him or her toward obtaining a job while in the rehabilitation program. The VR&E has stationed 83 Employment Coordinators (ECs) at regional VA offices across the country with the primary task of providing disabled veterans with any necessary job-readiness skills as well as job referral or placement services. Efforts have been made by the VA to increase employment opportunities for disabled veterans through partnerships with the Department of Labor, other federal agencies and organizations, and with employers across the nation.

CASE MANAGEMENT

A case manager is assigned to each recipient of VR&E services. The case manager works with a Vocational Rehabilitation Counselor (VRC) who must determine if, and why, the disabled veteran has experienced employability restrictions (or employment handicaps). A written rehabilitation plan must be developed by the VA and the veteran, describing the goal of the VR&E program and the means through which the goal will be achieved. The VRC will work with the veteran to assess his or her status and help to develop the written rehabilitation plan. The VRC and the case manager help the veteran to achieve the goals of the agreed upon written plan for employment or independent living. The VRC or case manager may provide referrals for medical and dental services, coordination of training allowances, tutorial assistance, or other services to achieve rehabilitation.

The rehabilitation phase of the VR&E program includes the following key components:

- evaluation and planning;
- extended evaluation;
- rehabilitation and employability (training or education);
- independent living;
- job ready status; and
- interrupted status.

Under the current VR&E program, a veteran whose eligibility and entitlement have been established must not only complete the rehabilitation plan, but he or she will also be tracked to attainment of suitable employment based on the plan's goals.

By law,[7] the VR&E services provided include the following:

- educational, personal, and psychological counseling and evaluation;
- vocational training benefits;
- loans;
- monthly subsistence allowance and work study allowance;
- medical benefits, including treatment, care, prosthetic appliances, and eyeglasses;
- any family support that is necessary to aid rehabilitation;
- case management services;
- travel and incidentals' allowance to defray costs of expenses incurred during rehabilitation, job seeking, and initial employment;
- special services related to blindness and deafness;
- assistance with independent living services;
- placement and employment services; and
- post placement services to ensure satisfactory adjustment in employment.

One of the task force's major recommendations led to the development of a new Five-Track Service Delivery System designed to make the VR&E's services more employment-driven. Veterans must choose one of the following five tracks to reach their employment goals: Re-employment; Rapid Access to Employment; Self-Employment; Employment through Long-Term Services; or Independent Living Services. The five tracks are described briefly below.

The Five-Track Service Delivery System

Re-Employment Track

The Re-employment Track helps veterans and members of the National Guard and the Reserves return to jobs held prior to active duty. Veterans, National Guard, and Reserve members may be provided with job accommodations, job modification, case management, coordination, and linkages to services with VA healthcare, re-employment rights advice, work adjustment services, and consultations with employers.

Rapid Access to Employment Track

The Rapid Access to Employment Track emphasizes the goal of immediate employment and is available to those who already have the skills to compete in the job market in appropriate occupations. Among other things, veterans may be provided job readiness preparation, resume development, job search assistance, and accommodations. ECs provide post-employment follow- up.

Self-Employment Track

This track is for veterans who have limited access to traditional employment and need flexible work schedules and a more accommodating work environment because of their disabling conditions or other special circumstances. Veterans may be provided an analysis of the viability of a business concept, development of a business plan, training in the operation of small businesses, marketing and financial assistance, and guidance on obtaining adequate resources to implement the business plan.

Employment through Long-Term Services Track

Under this track, the VR&E assists veterans who need specialized training or education to obtain and maintain suitable employment. Training or education (or both) may be provided, including on-the-job training, apprenticeships, internships, job shadowing, work monitoring, work-study, public-private job partnering, or higher education sufficient to obtain suitable entry-level employment.

Independent Living Services Track

The Independent Living Services Track is for veterans who may not be able to work immediately and need additional rehabilitation to enable them to live more independently. Veterans may be provided with assistive technology, independent living skills training, and connections to community-based support services.

The Independent Living (IL) Program is designed to help veterans whose service-connected disability or disabilities may be so severe that they are unable to immediately pursue an employment goal. It helps them to be able to live independently, participate in family and community life, and increase their potential to return to work. The IL program was established under P.L. 96-466, the Veterans Rehabilitation and Education Amendments of 1980, with an annual cap of 500 new cases per fiscal year. In succeeding years, the number of cases grew as the program's success in helping severely disabled veterans gain greater independence in daily living was recognized. The cap was increased by P.L. 107-103, the Veterans Education and Benefits Expansion Act of 2001, to 2,500 new cases per fiscal year. The Veterans' Benefits Improvement Act of 2008 (P.L. 110-389) further increased the cap to

2,600 new cases per fiscal year. The Veterans' Benefits Act of 2010 (P.L. 111-275) increased the cap to 2,700 for fiscal years beginning after enactment (FY20 12).

Program expenditures are generally capped at $25,000 per veteran per calendar year. For expenditures over this amount, the counselor must get approval from the local VR&E office. The Director of the VA Regional Office must approve costs exceeding $75,000 per veteran per calendar year. For program costs above $100,000 per veteran per calendar year and IL-related construction costs exceeding $25,000 per calendar year, approval must be sought from the Director of the VR&E Service.[8] IL programs for veterans are usually 24 months in duration, but they may be extended for an additional six months in exceptional circumstances. P.L. 110-389 provided a waiver from the 24-month limitation if the VA Secretary determines that additional time is need for a veteran with post 9/11 service who has a severe disability.

Assessment for participation in the IL program is done by counselors with specialized experience and training and is usually done in the veteran's home. The counselor works with the veteran to develop an IL plan that outlines the goals, services, and assistance to be provided and benchmarks to be used to determine progress in achieving greater independence in daily living. Services are tailored to the veteran's individual needs.

To meet the needs of veterans with severe disabilities and mobility impairments, VR&E's IL program works with the VA's Loan Guaranty Service and the Specially Adapted Housing (SAH) grant program,[9] the Home Improvements and Structural Alterations (HISA) program, the Automobile Adaptive Equipment program, and the Visually Impaired Services Team (VIST). The VR&E also works with the Committee on Care of Veterans with Severe Mental Illness (SMI)[10] and the Traumatic Brain Injury Caregivers Panel.[11]

IL program services may include the following:

- training in activities of daily living;
- attendant care during period of transition;
- transportation when special arrangements are required;
- assistive technology;
- specialized medical, health, and rehabilitation services;
- services to address any personal and/or family adjustment issues;
- peer counseling;
- housing integral to participation in a program of special rehabilitation services;
- training in independent living skills;
- connection with community-based support services;
- training to improve awareness of rights and needs;
- assistance in identifying and maintaining volunteer or supported employment;
- services to decrease social isolation; and
- adaptive equipment that increases functional independence.

A veteran eligible for the IL program must submit a completed application Form VA 28-1900 for VR&E services. He or she must also undergo a comprehensive evaluation by a counselor who will determine if the veteran is entitled to program services and if the IL program is appropriate for the veteran.

Vocational-Educational Counseling

The VR&E also provides a wide range of vocational-educational counseling to active duty servicemembers as well as to veterans and their dependents who are eligible for education benefits. [12] The VR&E program is distinct from the Montgomery GI Bill. [13] Servicemembers are eligible for these services six months prior to discharge from active duty or within one year after discharge. The services are designed to help these individuals choose a vocational direction and the course necessary to achieve their goals. Assistance may include testing for aptitude, exploring occupations, setting occupational goals, locating the right type of training program, and exploring educational or training facilities to achieve a vocational goal.

If a disabled veteran is enrolled in a vocational rehabilitation program, the VR&E pays the cost of tuition, fees, required books, supplies, and equipment. The VR&E may also pay for supportive services such as medical and dental care, prosthetic devices, lip-reading training, and signing for the deaf.

The goal of the education component of the VR&E program is to "address the continuum of 'life cycle' needs that a veteran with disabilities experiences, of which education may—or may not— be a necessary part. The focus will be the rehabilitation and employment needs of the 21st century service-connected disabled veteran."[14]

Veterans who need additional education or training to become employable are paid a subsistence allowance while they participate in vocational rehabilitation training. This subsistence allowance is larger than the stipend under the GI Bill program. It is based on whether training is part-time or full-time, the number of dependents, and the type of training.[15]

Children with Spina Bifida and Other Birth Defects

The VR&E provides services to children of Vietnam veterans who were born with Spina Bifida[16] or may have other covered birth defects. These children are entitled to receive vocational training, education, and employment services as well as other career-directed support services. These services generally last 24 months, but they may continue if the child has been unsuccessful in attaining suitable employment.

Services provided differ from those provided to veterans in the following ways. There is

- no subsistence allowance;
- no adaptation of automotive equipment;
- no extension of evaluation of employability beyond 30 days; and
- no independent living program.

Special Restorative Training

The VR&E may also provide special restorative training and counseling to eligible spouses and children[17] to help them to overcome or lessen mental or physical disabilities.

Once eligible, the spouse or children will receive a comprehensive evaluation to identify the best program or services for their needs. A case manager assists the family member throughout the entire program. The family member is also entitled to an accelerated educational assistance allowance for high tuition programs.[18] Normal assistance may continue until the spouse or child has achieved the goals of the special restorative training program.

The Coming Home to Work Program

The VR&E has established job resource labs in its regional offices, as well as an online employment resource known as VetSuccess.gov.[19] The Coming Home to Work (CHTW) program is VR&E's primary early intervention and outreach program. The goal of CHTW is to provide rehabilitation services to VR&E eligible servicemembers pending medical separation and to veterans receiving treatment at community-based health care organizations and VA medical treatment facilities.[20] CHTW is designed to help provide a seamless transition to VR&E services.[21]

VR&E eligible servicemembers with at least a 20% disability rating are entitled to an evaluation for VR&E benefits regardless of their expected discharge date.

Eligibility and Entitlement

Eligibility and entitlement must be established for participation in the VR&E program. A veteran who has an employment handicap and is eligible for the VR&E program is entitled to all applicable services. The program originally provided benefits to veterans with a 30% or more service-connected disability rating.[22] However, it has been modified to include veterans with a 10% or 20% disability rating.

Eligibility

To be considered eligible for VA benefits, a claimant must be a veteran or the survivor or dependent of a veteran. The services of the VR&E program are also available to active military personnel who are in medical-hold or pre-discharge status.[23] These individuals may be pre- qualified for the program.

To be eligible for VR&E services, a veteran must:

- have received, or will receive, a discharge under conditions other than dis-honorable;[24]
- have served on or after September 16, 1940;
- have a service-connected disability employment handicap rating of at least 20% or a serious employment handicap rating of 10%;
- need vocational rehabilitation to overcome an employment handicap; and
- submit a completed application for VR&E services on VA Form 28-1900.

Servicemembers pending medical separation from active duty may apply for VR&E services if their disabilities are reasonably expected to be rated at a minimum of at least 20% following their discharge. Each veteran must work with a case manager who will advise him or her on the series of steps to be taken to receive VR&E program services. The steps are described below:

Step 1. Application (described later in this chapter) for benefits and assessment of program eligibility.

Step 2. Evaluation to assess needs and determine services to which a veteran may be entitled, and formulation of a plan of rehabilitation.

Step 3. Provision of rehabilitation services for either employment (services and assistance that lead to the veteran becoming job-ready) or achievement of a measure of increased ability to live more independently in the community.

Step 4. Completion of the rehabilitation process. Veterans who have obtained and maintained suitable employment or achieved maximum independence in daily living are considered to be rehabilitated. *Suitable employment* is work within a veteran's physical and emotional capabilities and consistent with his or her patterns of abilities, aptitudes, and interests.

Entitlement

The VRC makes the entitlement determination on the basis of whether the veteran's employment problems have been caused by

- the veteran's service-connected disabilities;
- the veteran's non service-connected disabilities;
- deficiencies in education and training;
- negative attitudes about people with disabilities;
- the impact of alcoholism or drug abuse;
- consistency with abilities, aptitudes, and interests; or
- other pertinent factors.

To be entitled to vocational rehabilitation program services a veteran must be within the eligibility period (12 years) and have a disability rating of at least 20% with an employment handicap. Veterans with a disability rating of at least 10% with a serious employment handicap are entitled to program services regardless of whether the veteran is within the eligibility period.

What is an Employment Handicap?

An *employment handicap* as defined by law[25] is an impairment of a veteran's ability to prepare for, obtain, or retain employment consistent with his or her abilities, aptitudes, and interests. The impairment results in substantial part from a service-connected disability. Veterans with a disability rating of at least 20% and an employment handicap are entitled to VR&E program services.

What is a Serious Employment Handicap?

A *serious employment handicap* as defined by law[26] is a significant impairment of a veteran's ability to prepare for, obtain, or retain employment consistent with his or her abilities, aptitudes, and interests. The impairment results in substantial part from a service-connected disability. A disability rating of at least 10% and a serious employment handicap entitles a veteran to VR&E program services. If employment is not feasible, the veteran is evaluated for the Independent Living Program.

The primary difference between an employment handicap and a serious employment handicap is the degree of vocational impairment. The veteran's service-connected disability must contribute to the employment handicap. That is, the VR&E must be able to identify, observe, and measure it.

Certain totally disabled veterans are also eligible for VR&E program services. A veteran with a single disability rating of 60% or more, or a combined rating from more than one disability of at least 70%, where one disability is rated at 40% or higher, will be rated totally disabled for VR&E program purposes and be eligible for services.[27]

A veteran who is ineligible for VR&E services will be informed in person and will be sent a letter with information about appeal rights and the appeals process. The counselor will also use the information gathered in the application process to recommend other options, programs, or services that should contribute to the achievement of vocational adjustment. Other programs and services recommended may include State Vocational Rehabilitation programs and the Department of Labor's Disabled Veterans Outreach Program (DVOP).

Period of Eligibility

The period of eligibility for VR&E benefits is 12 years from (1) the date of separation from active military service or (2) the date the veteran was first notified by the VA of a service-connected disability rating.

The period of eligibility may be extended if the VRC determines that a veteran has a serious employment handicap, or has not yet been rehabilitated to the point of employability, or has been rehabilitated but still cannot perform the duties required, or needs more services because the occupational requirements have changed. An objective evaluation is required for these circumstances to be determined.

For independent living services, if the medical condition is so severe that achievement of the vocational goal is not feasible and that goal is necessary to ensure that the veteran will achieve maximum independence, the period of eligibility may be extended.

The Application Process

A veteran, his or her authorized representative, or a Member of Congress may communicate the veteran's intent to seek benefits under the VR&E program. The veteran must follow up by completing an application for the program. If the application is completed within one year of the communication of intent to file a claim, the date of the communication will be considered the date of formal application for benefits. The completion of applications is subject to time limits. Applications with missing information are returned for completion. The completed application must be returned within a year from the date of notification, or the veteran may be considered ineligible for benefits.[28]

The period from application to notification of entitlement averaged 48 days in FY2008.[29]

UTILIZATION OF VR&E SERVICES

For FY2006, the Office of Management and Budget (OMB) program performance measures noted that the VR&E program was making notable progress toward achieving long-term performance measures.[30] Data from the Department of Defense (DOD) used in the evaluations indicated that each year, approximately 25,000 active duty servicemembers are found "'not fit for duty' due to medical conditions that may qualify them for a VA disability rating and VR&E services."[31] During the evaluation, data from the Army Reserve and the Army National Guard indicated that 29,000 of their members had been placed on medical hold or extension status since 2003.[32] These servicemembers may qualify for VR&E services.

In FY2009, the VR&E spent $447.1 million on books, tuition, supplies, fees, and other costs for 17,400 program participants. In FY2009, VR&E spending on subsistence allowance benefits was $59.8 million for services to 59,829 recipients. In FY2009, VR&E provided rehabilitation, evaluation, planning, and services to 20,996 veterans or their dependents. No monetary benefit is associated with the latter services.[33]

For FY2008, OMB reported a rehabilitation rate of 76% for all disabled veterans in the VR&E program; the rehabilitation rate for serious employment handicaps was also reported to be 76%.[34]

Table 1. Vocational Rehabilitation & Employment Program Statistics, FY2008

VR&E Category	Total
Applicants	68,949
Eligible	65,784
Completed evaluation	39,910
Entitled to Services	35,166
Participants	103,126
Rehabilitated	11,039

Source: Table prepared by the Congressional Research Service (CRS) using data from the Department of Veterans Affairs, *Veterans Benefits Administration Annual Benefits Report, Fiscal Year 2006*, p. 62.

As shown in **Table 1**, in FY2008, from a pool of 68,949 applicants, 51.0% or 35,166 disabled veterans were found to be entitled to VR&E services, and there were 103,126 participants in the VR&E program.[35] The number of disabled veterans who were successfully rehabilitated by the end of the FY2008 program year was 11,039. Of this number, the number of veterans with serious employment handicaps that were rehabilitated in FY2008 was 6,146.[36]

The life cycle of one VR&E case may be four or more years from application to eligibility, entitlement, rehabilitation planning, achievement of rehabilitation goals, and finally, rehabilitation.

CURRENT ISSUES

The Supplemental Appropriations Act, 2008 (P.L. 110-252) included the Post-9/11 Veterans Educational Assistance Act of 2008. This new education benefit for veterans took effect August 1, 2009. Veterans participating in the vocation rehabilitation program could, if still eligible for benefits under the previous education benefit for veterans, the All-Volunteer Force Educational Assistance, have the education benefits paid through that program rather than through the vocational rehabilitation program. A similar option does not exist for veterans in the vocational rehabilitation program who are eligible for benefits under the new Post 9/11 education benefit program.[37]

OTHER EMPLOYMENT ASSISTANCE PROGRAMS FOR DISABLED VETERANS

Apart from the VR&E program, other federal agencies administer programs that provide services to help veterans to achieve an employment outcome, that is, to obtain competitive employment. VR&E has signed Memorandums of Understandings (MOUs) and formed partnerships with other organizations whose services frequently overlap, representing joint efforts to increase opportunities for rehabilitated veterans to become employed. In addition, each branch of the military has a program to support its disabled veterans, and many veterans service organizations (VSOs) provide services to disabled veterans, as well.

Listed below are some programs that provide rehabilitation or other services to veterans with brief descriptions and contact information. Links to many of these programs are provided from the VR&E program section of the VA website.

FEDERAL GOVERNMENT PROGRAMS

Computer/Electronics Accommodations Program

The Computer/Electronics Accommodations Program (CAP) provides assistive technology and services to people with disabilities, federal managers, supervisors, Internet technology (IT) professionals, and wounded servicemembers. Accommodations are made for servicemembers with vision or hearing loss, dexterity impairments (including upper-extremity amputees), and communication and cognitive difficulties, including Traumatic Brain Injuries (TBI). These services are available as a part of the DOD Military Health System's Tricare program. [38]

The Department of Education: Office of Special Education and Rehabilitative Services Administration

The Rehabilitative Services Administration (RSA) oversees grant programs that help individuals with mental or physical disabilities obtain employment and live more independently through the provision of such support as counseling, medical and psychological services, job training and other individualized services.

The Department of Labor

The Department of Labor's (DOL's) Veterans Employment and Training Services (VETS) falls under the President's National Hire Veterans Committee.[39] The mission of VETS is to provide veterans and transitioning servicemembers with the resources and services to succeed in the workforce by maximizing their employment opportunities, protecting their employment rights, and meeting labor market demands with qualified veterans. VETS administers the HireVetsFirst program to furnish employers with information about the training and skills of veterans and disabled veterans and the advantages afforded employers by hiring veterans with such training; and to provide a link to one stop centers and other employment job search assistance for veterans.[40]

The DOL also has a link from its website to a recruiting firm, RecruitMilitary, which focuses on matching military veterans and their spouses with employers around the world. RecruitMilitary lists more than 6,000 employers on its website.[41]

Disabled Transition Assistance Program

The VR&E partners with the DOD and the DOL through the Disabled Transition Assistance Program (DTAP) to allow disabled servicemembers to gain information and assistance with the transition from military to civilian life prior to their separation from military service.

The Compensated Work Therapy Program

The VR&E Compensated Work Therapy Program administered by the DOL brings transitional and permanent jobs to veterans who are returning to the workforce after medical rehabilitation. The program combines work and training for new job skills.[42]

The National Veterans Employment Program

The VA administers the National Veterans Employment Program (NVEP) to help veterans understand and use veterans' preference and other hiring flexibilities to get jobs in the federal government, including the VA. The program promotes the hiring of veterans by federal managers and supervisors. It also educates selecting officials on veterans' preference and federal hiring authorities developed to help veterans gain federal employment.[43]

The Office of Personnel Management

Most federal departments and agencies are required to have an affirmative action program for the recruitment, employment, and advancement of disabled veterans. Agencies develop Disabled Veterans Affirmative Action Programs (DVAAPs) and must submit accomplishment reports to the OPM reporting their efforts to promote the maximum employment and job advancement opportunities for disabled veterans. OPM provides guidance and assistance to agencies on the preparation of their DVAAPs and presents an annual report to Congress on the employment of veterans in the federal government.[44]

The Small Business Administration

In partnership with the Association of Small Business Development Centers (ASBDC), the Small Business Administration (SBA) provides entrepreneurial training to qualified service-connected disabled veterans who are VR&E participants. The mission of SBA's Office of Veterans Business Development is to maximize the availability, applicability, and usability of all SBA programs for veterans, service-disabled veterans, Reserve component members, and their dependents and survivors. The SBA provides grants to Veterans Business Outreach Center (VBOC) programs that assist disabled veterans with funding, counseling, mentoring, training, procurement, service delivery, business development, and government certification.[45]

Military Programs

Air Force Palace HART-Helping Airmen Recover together Program

The Air Force, through its Palace HART program, helps Air Force personnel who have been medically separated from active duty receive transition services by ensuring that they have complete information about entitlements that are due to them. When an airman enters the disability evaluation process, the Air Force Personnel Center begins tracking him or her for Palace HART eligibility. Once the airman is medically separated as a result of service-related injuries, Palace HART Family Support Centers provide transition services, including individual pre-separation counseling and assistance in obtaining all authorized service from the Air Force, the DOD, the VA, and the DOL. The program assists with the initial filing of VA disability claims, extended five-year case management follow-up, and employment placement assistance and counseling. The goal is to help wounded Air Force veterans transfer back to civilian life. [46]

Army Career and Alumni Program and Its Entrepreneurship Bootcamp for Veterans with Disabilities

Veterans disabled in support of Operations Iraqi Freedom and Enduring Freedom who are accepted into the Entrepreneurship Bootcamp for Veterans with Disabilities (EBV) program of the Army Career and Alumni Program (ACAP) can receive free training in entrepreneurship and small business management, as well as support in growing a successful business from the business school faculties of the following four U.S. universities: Whitman School of Management at Syracuse University; the College of Business at Florida State University; Anderson School of Management at the University of California at Los Angeles (UCLA); and Mays Business School at Texas A&M University. Eligible veterans may go online to apply for ACAP services.[47]

Army Material Command: Always a Soldier

The Always a Soldier program provides service-connected disabled veterans with opportunities to seek employment, career advancement, job mobility, family economic well-being, and greater financial security. Specific employment tracks include the following:

- federal wage grade positions involving trades and labor;
- internship programs providing monitored or supervised work or training experience with learning goals; and
- various federal general schedule (GS) series full performance positions.

The Always a Soldier program partners with existing Army programs (such as Disabled Soldier Services and Army Community Service), the VA, and the Disabled American Veterans (DAV) organization.[48]

Marine for Life-Injured Support Program

The goal of the Marine for Life-Injured Support (M4L-IS) Program is to provide needs-based individual support to combat-wounded marines and sailors from the time of injury through the post-discharge transition period (up to one year after release from active duty) until they are fully integrated into the VA system. The program's features include pre-and post-service separation case assistance; coordination with physical evaluation boards; coordination with veterans, public, and private organizations providing support to the seriously injured; and provision of referral services for disability specific information and mental health services.[49]

Navy Safe Harbor Program

The Navy Personnel Command website has links to a number of employment services for veterans and disabled veterans, including the DOL's Office of Disability Employment Program (ODEP) and State Vocational Rehabilitation Services.[50]

U.S. Army Wounded Warrior Program

The U.S. Army Wounded Warrior (AW2) program tracks soldiers and their families for five years after medical retirement. Army wounded warriors must suffer from injuries or illnesses incurred after September 11, 2001, in support of the Global War on Terror and receive a 30% disability rating[51] for one or more injuries.[52]

In response to the recommendations of the 2004 Task Force report, the VR&E has endeavored to develop an integrated working relationship with a wide range of organizations, such as the Centers for Independent Living; the National Council on Disability, the National Council on Independent Living, the Commission on Accreditation of Rehabilitation Facilities, and the National Organization of Disability Examining Physicians. The VR&E has also increased interaction with the vocational rehabilitation activities of academic organizations and private sector disability, rehabilitation, and employment firms and associations.

The VR&E maintains strategic partnerships with private sector companies such as the Home Depot, the Mortgage Bankers Association, and faith-based organizations such as the YMCA, Goodwill Industries International, and Disabled Sports to achieve the goal of integrated and seamless delivery of services to disabled veterans.

End Notes

[1] The other four are compensation and pension, life insurance, education, and loan guaranty.

[2] The term employment handicap is defined by law in 38 U.S.C. §3101.

[3] The VR&E program is authorized under 38 U.S.C. Chapter 31.

[4] Congressional Commission on Servicemembers and Veterans Transition Assistance, *Congressional Commission on Servicemembers and Veterans Transition Assistance,* January 1999, pp. 84-85, available at http://www.va.gov/vetbiz/ library/Transition%20Commission%20Report.pdf.

[5] U.S. Department of Veterans Affairs, VA Vocational Rehabilitation and Employment Task Force, *Report to the Secretary of Veterans Affairs: The Vocational Rehabilitation and Employment Program for the 21st Century Veteran, 2004*, hereinafter referred to as the VR&E Task Force Report, available at http://w ww1.va.gov/op3/docs/ VRE_Report.pdf.

[6] U.S. Department of Veterans Affairs, *FY2007 Performance and Accountability Report*, November 15, 2007, Part I, p. 55, available at http://www.va.gov/budget/report/2007/index.htm.

[7] 38 U.S.C. § 3100, § 3104, § 3109, and § 3120.

[8] Testimony of Ruth Fanning, Director, VA's VR&E Service, before the House Committee on Veterans' Affairs, Subcommittee on Economic Opportunity, *Independent Living Program,* 110th Cong., 2nd Sess., July 10, 2008.

[9] For information on housing and automobile grants, see CRS Report RL34626, *Veterans' Benefits: Benefits Available for Disabled Veterans*, by Christine Scott and Carol D. Davis.

[10] The 2004 VR&E Task Force Report noted "that the single largest group of veterans for whom an employment plan is not considered feasible was for veterans with psychiatric disabilities," p. A-64.

[11] P.L. 110-181, signed by President George W. Bush on January 28, 2008, mandated the creation of the Traumatic Brain Injury Caregivers Panel to develop coordinated, uniform, and consistent training curricula to be used in training family members in the provision of care and assistance to current and former members of the Armed Forces with traumatic brain injury. For details see CRS Report RL34371, *"Wounded Warrior" and Veterans*

Provisions in the FY2008 National Defense Authorization Act, by Sarah A. Lister, Christine Scott, and Sidath Viranga Panangala

[12] Dependents are eligible for benefits under 38 U.S.C. Chapters 18, 32, 30, and 35.

[13] See CRS Report R40723, *Educational Assistance Programs Administered by the U.S. Department of Veterans Affairs*, by Cassandria Dortch.

[14] The VR&E Task Force Report, p. 165.

[15] For current rates see the Department of Veterans Affairs rate tables, available at http://www.vba.va.gov/bln/vre/doc/ sa_rates.pdf.

[16] 38 U.S.C. Chapter 18.

[17] 38 U.S.C. Chapter 35.

[18] The monthly rate of $788 is for special restorative training that occurs after June 30, 2004 in accordance with 38 U.S.C. 3542 38 C.F.R. 21.3333 (a)(1).

[19] Available at http://www.vetsuccess.gov.

[20] The Community Based Health Care Organization (CBHCO) Program was created to assist Guard and Reserve servicemembers injured in the line of duty to return to their homes where they will continue to receive medical care locally while they are evaluated for return to duty, medical release, or medical board. To be eligible, the servicemember must have a referral into the program from their respective branch of service. National Guard and Reserve servicemembers must agree to remain on active duty status to be enrolled in the CBHCO program.

[21] To apply for Coming Home To Work services, servicemembers without a VA disability rating must complete VA Form 28-0588,*Vocational Rehabilitation and Employment - Getting Ahead After You Get Out*, and submit it with medical records and a completed application for VR&E services (VA Form 28-1900) to the nearest VA regional office.

[22] For more information about the VA rating system, see CRS Report RL33323, *Veterans Affairs: Benefits for Service- Connected Disabilities*, by Douglas Reid Weimer.

[23] For a description of medical hold discharge status, see CRS Report RL33991, *Disability Evaluation of Military Servicemembers*, by Christine Scott and Don J. Jansen.

[24] For more information on discharge criteria, see CRS Report RL33 113, *Veterans Affairs: Basic Eligibility for Disability Benefit Programs*, by Douglas Reid Weimer.

[25] 38U.S.C. §3101, (1).

[26] 38 U.S.C. §3 101, (2).

[27] These veterans are awarded total disability benefits (compensation) based on individual unemployability, and are afforded VR&E benefits.

[28] Applications may be submitted online or by mail. Online applications are available on the VA website at http://vabenefits.vba.va.gov/vonapp/main.asp. Applications filed online go directly to the appropriate VA office. Applications that will be mailed in must be submitted on VA Form 28-1900, *Disabled Veterans Application for Vocational Rehabilitation*. The form can be downloaded from the VA website at http://www.va.gov/vaforms, or veterans may call 1-800-827-1000 and request that the form be sent to them by mail. The completed form should be mailed to the nearest VA Regional Office. There are 57 VA regional offices that carry out the functions of the Veterans Benefits Administration. To identify the nearest office, veterans should go to http://www1.va.gov/directory/guide/ home.asp.

[29] Available at http://www.whitehouse.gov/omb/expectmore/detail/10003220.2006.html.

[30] Ibid.

[31] Ibid.

[32] Ibid.

[33] U.S. Department of Veterans Affairs: *FY2009 Budget Submission: Benefits and Burial Programs and Departmental Administration*, Vol. 3 of 4, February 2008, pp.2A2-2A3, available at http://www.va.gov/budget/summary/2009/ Volume_3-Benefits_and_Burial_and_Dept_Admin.pdf.

[34] Available at http://www.whitehouse.gov/omb/expectmore/detail/1003220.2006.html.

[35] Participants are veterans who are receiving a subsistence allowance in one of the following case statuses: extended evaluation, independent living, job ready, or rehabilitation to employment.

[36] "Rehabilitated" means veterans who have successfully found and maintained suitable employment or have successfully completed an independent living program.

[37] For more information on new education benefit see CRS Report R40723, *Educational Assistance Programs Administered by the U.S. Department of Veterans Affairs*, by Cassandria Dortch.

[38] Available at http://tricare.mil/cap/wsm/.

[39] Jobs for Veterans Act (P.L. 107-288); currently codified at 38 U.S.C. § 4100.

[40] Available at http://www.dol.gov/vets/ and http://www.hirevetsfirst.gov.

[41] Available at http ://recruitmilitary. com.

[42] Available at http://www1.va.gov/Vetind/.

[43] Available at http://www.va.gov/nvep/.

[44] Available at http://www.opm.gov/veterans/dvaap.asp.

[45] Available at http://www.sba.gov/aboutsbs/sbaprograms/ovbd/index.html.
[46] Available at http://www.af.mil.
[47] Available at http://acap.army.mil and http://www.acapexpress.army.mil.
[48] Available at http://www.amc.army.mil/alwaysasoldier.
[49] Available at http://www.mfl.usmc.mil.
[50] See http://www.npc.navy.mil/CommandSupport/SafeHarbor/SH_JobPlacement.htm.
[51] Conditions are based on the VA Schedule for Disability Ratings (VASDR) 2003 C.F.R. 38 Chapter 1, Part 4 as used by the U.S. Army Physical Disability Agency (USPDA).
[52] Available at http://www.aw2.army.mil.

In: Veterans Benefits
Editors: George B. Meyers and Alice M. Glaskin
ISBN: 978-1-61209-581-3

Chapter 10

EDUCATIONAL ASSISTANCE PROGRAMS ADMINISTERED BY THE U.S. DEPARTMENT OF VETERANS AFFAIRS

Cassandria Dortch

SUMMARY

The U.S. Department of Veterans Affairs (VA), previously named the Veterans Administration, has been providing veterans educational assistance benefits since 1944. The benefits have been intended, at various times, to compensate for compulsory service, encourage voluntary service, avoid unemployment, provide equitable benefits to all who served, and promote military retention. The categories of individuals eligible to receive benefits has expanded from just veterans to include service members, Reservists, National Guard members, and their dependents. Although the programs are administered by the VA, the Department of Defense pays certain benefits and provides additional benefits to certain persons with critical skills or lengthy service.

As of August 2009, there are six benefit programs available to eligible individuals who pursue education or training. A few veterans who first entered active duty service between December 31, 1976, and July 1, 1985, are still receiving benefits under the Post-Vietnam Era Veterans' Educational Assistance Program (VEAP). The program provides veterans a monthly subsistence allowance, which is equivalent to three times the service members' contribution over the life of the benefit, up to 36 months.

Other benefits are also available. The Montgomery GI Bill has a program for individuals with active duty service known as the Montgomery GI Bill-Active Duty (MGIB-AD), and a program with lower benefit payments for Reservists known as the Montgomery GI Bill-Selected Reserves (MGIB-SR). To become eligible for the MGIB-AD, most service members must make a $1,200 contribution; however, the benefit amount is not related to the contribution. To remain eligible for the MGIB-SR, the individual must remain on active duty or in the Reserves. The Reserves Educational Assistance Program (REAP) provides benefits to Reservists with active duty service. The benefit levels are higher than the MGIB-SR but lower than the MGIB-AD.

The newest program, the Post-9/11 GI Bill, started providing benefits on August 1, 2009. Many individuals currently eligible for the MGIB-AD and REAP are also be eligible for the Post-9/11 GI Bill. The program is designed to provide veterans who choose to attend public colleges and universities for their undergraduate studies with the full cost of attendance: tuition and fees, housing allowance, books and supplies stipend, tutorial and relocation assistance, and fees for a testing and certification, as needed. Individuals who attend private institutions of higher learning or public graduate and professional programs may receive additional benefits to cover a portion of their costs.

Finally, the dependents of individuals with military service may be eligible for four educational assistance programs. The Survivors' and Dependents' Educational Assistance (DEA) program provides benefits to the spouse and children of service members who, as a result of service, are seriously disabled, die, or are detained. The Army allows service members who stay in the military for several additional years to transfer their MGIB-AD benefits to their dependents. Service members who stay in the military for several years are able to transfer their Post-9/11 GI Bill benefits to their dependents. Also, the Post-9/11 GI Bill includes a scholarship program for the children of service members who die in the line of duty, the Marine Gunnery Sergeant John David Fry Scholarship Program.

INTRODUCTION

This chapter provides a detailed description of the six educational assistance programs that are available to veterans or other eligible individuals through the Department of Veterans Affairs (VA). Although the programs are administered by the VA, some of the funding for the programs is provided by the Department of Defense (DOD).[1] DOD transfers monies from its education trust fund to the VA for disbursement.

The report is organized into five sections. The first section provides an explanation of the rationale and impetus behind veterans' educational assistance programs (GI Bills). The second section describes the eligibility requirements and uses of the existing GI Bills. The third section reviews the linkages and commonalities between the programs. A summary of selected characteristics of the various programs is presented in **Table 3**. The fourth section provides a brief overview of related VA programs. The final section provides information on participation and expenditures for the programs. A detailed look at the earlier GI Bills, which have been repealed, is available in the appendices.

Over the decades during which the programs have been in existence, two themes have been emphasized. The benefits promote development of work related skills to facilitate entry or reentry into the workforce, and the base benefit is equitable regardless of rank or military occupation specialty. Educational assistance programs offered by DOD are targeted to specific skills or individuals. All of the educational assistance programs administered by the VA require some period of military service before benefits can be received. The most salient ongoing conflicts have been related to how much eligible individuals should contribute to their education in time or money, which type of service warrants a benefit, and how liberal (i.e., valuable) the benefit should be.

Table 1. Chronology of Educational Assistance Programs Administered by the VA

Year Enacted	Common Name	Establishing Legislation	U.S. Code
1944	Original GI Bill	Serviceman's Readjustment Act of 1944	Title 38, Chapter 12
1952	Korean Conflict GI Bill	Veterans' Readjustment Assistance Act of 1952	Title 38, Chapter 33 (repealed in 1966)
1966	Post-Korean Conflict and Vietnam Era GI Bill	Veterans Readjustment Benefits Act of 1966	Title 38, Chapter 34
1956	DEA (Survivors' and Dependents Educational Assistance)	War Orphans' Educational Assistance Act of 1956	Title 38, Chapter 35
1974	Veterans and Dependents Education Loan Program	Veterans' Readjustment Assistance Act of 1974	Title 38, Chapter 36 (repealed in 1981)
1976	VEAP (Post-Vietnam Era Veterans Educational Assistance)	Veterans' Education and Employment Assistance Act of 1976	Title 38, Chapter 32
1981	Educational Assistance Test Program (Sec. 901)	Department of Defense Authorization Act, 1981	Title 10, Chapter 106A
1981	Educational Assistance Pilot Program (Sec. 903)	Department of Defense Authorization Act, 1981	Title 10, Chapter 106A
1985	MGIB-AD (Montgomery GI Bill-Active Duty)	Department of Defense Authorization Act, 1985	Title 38, Chapter 30
1985	MGIB-SR (Montgomery GI Bill-Selected Reserves)	Department of Defense Authorization Act, 1985	Title 10, Chapter 1606
2005	REAP (Reserves Educational Assistance Program)	Ronald W. Reagan National Defense Authorization Act for FY2005	Title 10, Chapter 1607
2008	Post-9/11 GI Bill	Post-9/11 Veterans Educational Assistance Act of 2008	Title 38, Chapter 33
2009	Marine Gunnery Sergeant John David Fry Scholarship	Supplemental Appropriations Act of 2009 (P.L. 111-32)	Title 38, Chapter 33

Source: Prepared by CRS based on a review of the legislation.

All of the benefit programs provide eligible persons an *entitlement* to educational assistance. This entitlement is measured in dollars and/or time. Educational assistance payments reduce the total dollars of entitlement at a one-for-one basis; they also reduce the entitlement period at rates prescribed by Congress or in proportion to the base payment. Eligible persons may run out of dollars of entitlement before running out of the entitlement period or vice versa. Once either runs out, the total *entitlement* is exhausted. In general, once the entitlement period or dollars of entitlement are exhausted eligible persons continue receiving educational assistance through the end of the academic term if more than halfway through, or a 12-week period if not on an academic term schedule. Neither the entitlement period nor the dollars of entitlement are reduced if an individual is called to active duty under sections 12301(a), 12301(d), 12301(g), 12302, or 12304 of Title 10 U.S.C. and if, as a result, the individual must discontinue studies and fails to receive credit or training time.

HISTORY OF THE PROGRAMS

Since the Revolutionary War, the United States has provided benefits to injured or disabled war veterans; however, benefits were not provided to the same extent to their able-bodied peers. Prior to World War II (WWII), "poor, jobless, and disgruntled veterans ... had led to unrest and fear of revolt throughout American history." In 1932, after World War I, the military was called in to forcibly remove 20,000 still unemployed and often homeless veterans and burn their encampment near the Capitol and White House.[2]

Despite the draft, military service was thought of as "a fundamental obligation of [male] citizenship."[3] Because the 16.1 million personnel[4] who served in the U.S. Armed Forces[5] during WWII accounted for over one-third of the 41.1 million[6] working-age males (between 20 and 64 years of age) in 1947, fears of the consequences of mass unemployment were legitimate. Before the end of WWII, Congress and the American Legion[7] worked together to pass the original GI Bill, or Serviceman's Readjustment Act of 1944 (P.L. 78-346). The act provided a full range of resources to veterans including the construction of additional hospitals; educational assistance to non-disabled veterans; home, business, and farm loans; job counseling and employment placement services; and an unemployment benefit.

The original GI Bill was generally considered successful in averting unemployment, raising the educational level and thus the productivity of the U.S. workforce, and confirming the value that Americans place on those that provide military service. Subsequent GI Bills providing educational assistance have been passed (**Table 1**). The Korean Conflict GI Bill was enacted under the Veterans' Readjustment Assistance Act of 1952 (P.L. 82-550) and codified in Title 38, U.S.C., Chapter 33. The purpose of the program was to prepare returning veterans to enter the workforce. It allowed the same types of education and training as the original GI Bill—on-the-job training, on-the-farm training, correspondence courses,[8] and traditional college education. Several provisions were also added to prevent avocational or recreational educational pursuits and to ensure the quality of education provided.

The Post-Korean Conflict and Vietnam Era GI Bill was enacted under the Veterans Readjustment Benefits Act of 1966 (P.L. 89-358) and codified in Title 38, U.S.C., Chapter 34. In addition to providing benefits to veterans, it provided benefits to active duty service members to encourage retention in the armed forces. The Veterans' Readjustment Assistance Act of 1974 (P.L. 93-508) created a short-lived veterans and dependents education loan program to cover educational costs not provided for under the GI Bill. It was codified in Title 38, U.S.C., Chapter 36 before being repealed in 1981.

In 1956, the War Orphans' Educational Assistance Act of 1956 (P.L. 84-634) was passed to provide educational assistance to the children of service members who died as a result of injury or disability incurred in the line of duty. This program was later expanded to include spouses and children of service members who died, became permanently or totally disabled, were missing-inaction, were captured, or were hospitalized as a result of service. Most recently, through the Post- 9/11 GI Bill, educational assistance benefits are available to a spouse and children under certain circumstances.

Beginning with the Korean Conflict GI Bill, there has been much debate on the level of educational assistance that should be provided to veterans and service members. Some believed that requiring individuals to make a monetary contribution in addition to their military service would increase their sense of responsibility and purpose. Some believed that the educational assistance benefits were a necessary compensation for compulsory service or reimbursement for voluntary service. Some believed that high levels of assistance promote attrition from the military. And some believed that the benefits are a necessary recruitment tool.

Congress allowed the compulsory military draft to expire on June 30, 1973. The educational assistance programs enacted subsequently were designed to encourage recruitment and retention of high-quality military personnel while still providing a considerable benefit to those who choose to leave active duty military service. Since 1973, there has also been a consistent attempt to limit the options to a more traditional college education; although, other types of education and training are generally added as the programs mature.

Currently, five educational assistance programs are available to veterans and service members, and two are available to spouses and children. The oldest of these programs for veterans and service members is the Post-Vietnam Era GI Bill enacted in 1976. Several hundred individuals are still receiving benefits from this program, which provides educational assistance in direct proportion to contributions deducted from service members' pay while on active duty. The Montgomery GI Bill-Active Duty requires most service members to contribute an established amount, although the eventual benefits are not related to the contribution. The Montgomery GI Bill-Selected Reserves (MGIB-SR) only provides educational assistance to those currently serving in the Selected Reserves. Because reliance on the Reserves and National Guard increased after September 11, 2001, the Reserves Educational Assistance Program enacted in 2005 allows Reservists to receive an increased educational assistance benefit in comparison to the MGIB-SR after serving on active duty. Finally, the Post-9/11 GI Bill, effective August 1, 2009, increases the educational assistance benefit for all individuals with active duty service after September 10, 2001, in recognition that the United States has not been at peace since 2001. The following section describes in greater detail the active programs.

ACTIVE EDUCATIONAL ASSISTANCE PROGRAMS

Post-Vietnam Era Veterans Educational Assistance Program (VEAP)

The Post-Vietnam Era Veterans' Educational Assistance Program (VEAP) was established under Title IV of the Veterans' Education and Employment Assistance Act of 1976 (P.L. 94-502) and codified in Title 38, U.S.C., Chapter 32. The program was established to make education affordable and recruit qualified service members. VEAP was designed as a recruitment incentive for the Armed Forces during peacetime.[9]

Eligible Individuals

VEAP was the first GI Bill to make educational benefits available to both active duty and reserve components simultaneously from the outset. The Post-Korean Conflict GI Bill (see **Appendix C**) was amended to include Reservists who served on active duty for over a year. Under VEAP, educational assistance benefits are available to individuals who entered active duty after December 31, 1976, and before July 1, 1985. To be eligible for benefits, veterans must have been discharged or released other than dishonorably and must have served a minimum of 180 days of active duty, or they must have been discharged or released for a service-connected disability. Service members remaining in service must have completed their first obligated period of active duty[10] or six years of active duty, whichever is less. The 1 80-day active duty service period excludes time assigned to an education or training program similar to those offered to civilians, excludes time spent as a cadet or midshipman at one of the service academies, and excludes periods of receiving an allowance from the College First Program (10 U.S.C. § 511(d)) for a delayed enlistment in the Army National Guard or the Air National Guard or while a member of the Reserves.

Individuals eligible for the prior GI Bill, the Post Korean Conflict GI Bill (see **Appendix C**), are not eligible under VEAP, with one exception. Members of the National Guard[11] or Reserves who participated in the College First Program and who served at least one consecutive year of active duty after completing the period of active duty for training are eligible. The individual must make an irrevocable decision to receive benefits under VEAP.

Since the benefit was established for an all-volunteer force serving during peacetime, it was deemed appropriate to require participants to contribute to their educational fund during their period of service in the military. Program participants had to agree to monthly pay deductions of at least $25, but not more than $100, for a total contribution of up to $2,700.[12] After making at least 12 contributions, individuals could withdraw from the program, receiving their contributions in return and making them ineligible for program benefits.[13] The U.S. Department of Defense (DOD), as a recruitment or retention incentive, could also contribute additional monies, called "Kickers," into an individual's educational fund or contribute in lieu of the service member.

Benefit Availability and Duration of Use

Veterans and service members must use their educational assistance benefits within ten years of discharge or release from active duty. [14]

Under all of the GI bills, individuals are entitled to receive benefits over a maximum period of time (e.g., 36 or 48 months). Under VEAP, individuals are entitled to a maximum of 36 months (or the equivalent for part-time attendance) or the number of months in which contributions were made, whichever is less. Veterans and service members can combine benefits with other VA administered educational assistance programs to receive up to 48 months of educational benefits, but benefits cannot be received concurrently, and the eligibility periods cannot overlap.

Eligible Programs of Education, Institutions, and Establishments

The VEAP allows veterans and service members to attend a wide array of educational institutions and training establishments. Eligible educational institutions are

- public or private elementary or secondary schools;
- vocational, correspondence, business, normal, or professional schools;
- colleges or universities;
- scientific or technical institutions,
- other institutions furnishing education for adults;
- state-approved alternative teacher certification program providers;
- private entities that offer courses toward the attainment of a license or certificate generally recognized as necessary for a profession or vocation in a high technology occupation; and
- qualified providers of entrepreneurship courses.

Eligible training establishments are

- providers of apprentice or other on-the-job training;
- providers of self-employment on-the-job training that is needed or accepted to be licensed to engage in a self-employment occupation or to own and operate a franchise;
- a state board of vocational education;
- a federal or state apprenticeship registration agency;
- the sponsor of a program of apprenticeship; and
- an agency of the federal government authorized to supervise such training.

The eligible programs of education or educational expenditures are

- courses which lead to the attainment of a predetermined educational, vocational, or professional objective or objectives if related to the same career (this includes traditional undergraduate and graduate programs);
- courses which lead to a high school diploma;
- courses required by the Administrator of the Small Business Administration as a condition to obtaining financial assistance under the provisions of section 7(i)(1) of the Small Business Act (15 U.S.C. 636(i)(1));
- licensing or certification tests for a predetermined vocation or profession, provided such tests and the licensing or credentialing organizations or entities that offer such tests are approved;
- courses offered by a qualified provider of entrepreneurship courses;
- national tests for admission to institutions of higher learning or graduate schools (such as the Scholastic Aptitude Test (SAT));
- national tests providing an opportunity for course credit at institutions of higher learning (such as the Advanced Placement (AP) exam);
- full-time programs of apprentice or other on-the-job training; and
- cooperative programs[15] for individuals not on active duty.[16]

Benefit Payments

The VEAP benefit consists of a monthly allowance for subsistence, tuition and fees, supplies, books, and equipment paid directly to recipients while enrolled in training or a program of education. Individuals are entitled to three times their contribution plus any DOD contributions. The maximum monthly basic educational benefit may not exceed $300.[17] The entitlement period of individuals taking correspondence courses is reduced one month for each month of assistance regardless of the rate of attendance. Individuals incarcerated for a felony conviction in a federal, state, local, or other penal institution or correctional facility may only receive an allowance to cover actual tuition and fees and necessary supplies, books, and equipment.[18] Individuals in a program of education consisting exclusively of flight training receive 60% of the program's established charges. [19] Individuals may receive up to $2,000 for each licensing or certification test taken, and individuals may receive the actual fee for each admissions or course credit test taken.[20] For an individual in apprentice or on-the-job training, the monthly allowance is 75%, 55%, and 35% of the monthly benefit otherwise payable to that individual for the first six months, second six months, and thereafter, respectively.[21]

Individuals are also eligible for payments of up to $100 monthly (for a maximum of $1,200 total) for tutorial assistance. The individual must be enrolled at least half-time, and the educational institution must certify as to the necessity and customary nature of the cost. The first $600 does not reduce the entitlement period; however, the subsequent $600 reduces the entitlement period by one month for each amount paid, which is equal to the monthly benefit otherwise payable to that individual.

Montgomery GI Bill

House hearings examining the possible need for a new GI Bill in the early 1980s focused on the difficulties the military was experiencing in recruiting and retaining a highly qualified all- volunteer force: active duty, Reserves, and National Guard.[22] Although recruiting problems were not uniformly distributed by branch, rank, grade, or military occupational specialty (MOS), some suggested reinstating the draft. DOD was concerned by the high cost of attrition: training new recruits and loss of experience and expertise. Some witnesses argued for the elimination of the service member's contribution because retention rates were not appreciably increased by VEAP. Only 20-25% of new recruits contributed to VEAP, and 40% had disenrolled from the program to recoup their contribution, which equaled 5% to 20% of the after-tax pay for some enlisted members. Despite a strong desire to increase retention by allowing universal transfer of dollars of entitlement and the entitlement period to spouses and children after ten years of service, such a proposal was deemed too expensive.[23]

Montgomery GI Bill—Active Duty (MGIB-AD)

The Montgomery GI Bill-Active Duty (MGIB-AD), originally called the All-Volunteer Force Educational Assistance Program, was initially enacted as part of the Department of Defense Authorization Act, 1985 (P.L. 98-525), as a three-year pilot program.[24] The program was finally codified in Title 38, U.S.C., Chapter 30. The original purpose of the permanent program was to provide educational readjustment assistance and to aid in the recruitment and retention of highly qualified personnel for both the active and reserve components of the Armed Forces. It was also expected to promote and assist the All-Volunteer Force program and the Total Force Concept of the Armed Forces[25] based upon service on active duty or a combination of service on active duty and in the Selected Reserve, including the National Guard. To ensure the recruitment of higher quality individuals, more likely to stay in the military, the program requires that all individuals complete a high school diploma, its equivalent, or 12 credit hours of postsecondary education in order to be eligible for benefits.[26]

Eligible Individuals

Educational assistance benefits are available to four categories of individuals.

- **Category 1** individuals entered active-duty for the first time after June 30, 1985, and served a minimum of three continuous years on active duty, or two continuous years if the initial obligated period of active duty was less than three years. Category 1 individuals may also have been discharged with a service- connected disability, hardship, pre-existing condition, certain reductions-in-force, a physical or mental condition that did not result from the individual's own willful misconduct, or for the government's convenience after serving a minimum of 30 months active duty, or 20 months if the initial obligated period of active duty was less than three years. Category 1 individuals also include Selected Reservists and National Guard members who serve two continuous years of honorable active duty service upon first entry into the military after June 30, 1985, and who serve a minimum of four continuous years of service in the Reserves immediately following the active duty service. For Reservists and National Guard members, the active duty service period includes only Active Guard/Reserve duty under section 12103(d) of Title 10 U.S.C. and certain full- time National Guard duty for the purpose of organizing, administering, recruiting, instructing, or training the National Guard under Title 32 U.S.C. For Reservists and National Guard members, the active duty service period excludes time during which the individual was ordered to perform under section 12301, 12302, 12304, 12306, or 12307 of Title 10 U.S.C. for a period of less than two years. Commissioned officers of the Public Health Service (PHS) and the National Oceanic Atmospheric Association (NOAA) are also eligible.
- **Category 2** individuals had a remaining period of entitlement under the Post- Korean Conflict GI Bill (see **Appendix C**) as of December 31, 1989, and were on active duty after June 30, 1985.[27] Category 1 and 2 individuals exclude officers commissioned upon graduation from the U.S. Military, Naval, Air Force, or Coast Guard Academy after December 31, 1976. Category 1 and 2 individuals also exclude officers who complete training as cadets and midshipmen if the officer entered active duty before October 1, 1996, or entered active duty after September 30, 1996, and received more than $3,400 for each year of such participation.
- **Category 3** individuals elected MGIB-AD before receiving an involuntary separation, voluntary separation incentive, or special separation benefit.
- **Category 4** individuals are VEAP participants who either had a remaining period of entitlement; were on active duty on October 9, 1996; or elected to transfer to the MGIB-AD by October 9, 1997; and made the requisite $1,200 contribution. VEAP participants who served on active duty from October 9, 1996, through April 1, 2000; elected to transfer to the MGIB-AD by October 31, 2001; and made a $2,700 contribution are also in Category 4. A small group of National Guard members who

first served on full-time National Guard active duty under Title 32 U.S.C. between June 30, 1985, and November 29, 1989, were eligible to make the requisite $1,200 contribution during an open period from October 9, 1996, to June 8, 1997.

The active duty service period requirements exclude time assigned to an education or training program similar to those offered to civilians unless assigned by the military full-time, exclude time spent as a cadet or midshipman at one of the service academies, and exclude the initial 12- week period of active duty for training in the National Guard and Reserves. The active duty service period requirements include time spent organizing, administering, recruiting, instructing, or training the National Guard while on full-time Army National Guard or Air National Guard duty and include time spent at a service academy or preparing to attend a service academy if the individual fails and returns to active duty. Individuals in all categories must have completed a high school diploma, its equivalent, or 12 semester hours in a program of education leading to a standard college degree. Also, all individuals must continue on active duty or in the Reserves, as appropriate; be discharged under fully honorable conditions; be placed on the retired or temporary disability retired list; or be transferred to certain Reserve components.

To become eligible for MGIB-AD benefits, Category 1 individuals must not decline the benefit in writing, and must allow the first 12 months of their military pay to be reduced by $100 per month.[28] This is in contrast to the Post-Vietnam Era GI Bill, which required service members to elect to participate by making contributions. In certain circumstances, service members who initially declined the benefit were allowed to enroll in the program.[29] As with the Post-Vietnam GI Bill, to discourage experienced personnel from leaving the military, service members remaining in service are eligible to receive educational benefits; however, the period of service was reduced to allow benefits after serving just two continuous years on active duty (the VEAP requires completing the first obligated period of active duty or six years of active duty, whichever is less).

Benefit Availability and Duration

By law, no educational benefits under the MGIB-AD can be paid more than ten years after discharge or release from active duty, or in the case of a Reservist, more than ten years after completing the required four-year Selected Reserve duty.[30] Most individuals are entitled to 36 months (or the equivalent in part-time attendance) of educational assistance. Category 1 active duty service members discharged or released (other than for the convenience of the government) before serving the minimum two or three years of active duty service are entitled to educational benefits for a period equal to one month for each month of active duty service, but no more than 36 months. Reservists are entitled to one month for each month of active duty service and one month for each four months served in the Selected Reserves, but no more than 36 months.[31] Veterans and service members can combine benefits with other VA administered educational assistance programs to receive up to 48 months of education benefits, but benefits cannot be received concurrently, and the eligibility periods cannot overlap.

Eligible Programs of Education, Institutions, and Establishments

The list of eligible training establishments and educational institutions mirrors that of the Post- Vietnam Era GI Bill. The eligible programs of education are the same as the Post-

Vietnam Era GI Bill except that only non-active duty service members may enroll in apprentice or on-the-job training. Individuals may also enroll in preparatory courses for an admissions test to an institution of higher education (IHE) or graduate school.

Benefit Payments

Like the Post-Vietnam GI Bill, an allowance for subsistence, tuition and fees, supplies, books, and equipment is paid directly to recipients. Beginning with FY20 10, and unless Congress changes the amount, the maximum monthly benefit amounts will be adjusted annually based on the annual percentage increase in the average cost of undergraduate tuition in the United States, as determined by the National Center for Education Statistics (NCES).[32] The most recently published data from NCES shows that the average rates for in-state undergraduate tuition and required fees at public institutions for full-time students in degree-granting institutions increased 4.8%, from $4,102 in academic year 2006-2007 to $4,307 in academic year 2007-2008.[33] Effective October 1, 2009, veterans may receive up to $1,368 monthly for full-time training.[34] A reduced allowance is provided for less than full-time training and for those who served less than three years of active duty. Individuals on active duty and those training less than half-time receive actual tuition and fees or the monthly allowance, whichever is less. For an individual in apprentice or on-the-job training, the monthly allowance is 75%, 55%, and 35% of the monthly benefit otherwise payable to that individual for the first six months, second six months, and thereafter, respectively.[35] Individuals in cooperative training receive 80% of the monthly allowance.[36] Individuals pursuing education exclusively by correspondence receive 55% of the institution's established charges for completed courses, and individuals pursuing education consisting exclusively of flight training receive 60% of the institution's established charges for completed courses.[37]

Individuals may receive an accelerated payment of the basic educational assistance for education leading to employment in a high technology occupation in a high technology industry. If the costs of the program of education are more than double the monthly assistance allowance to which the individual would have been entitled, the individual may receive the lesser of 60% of the program's costs for the term or the individual's remaining dollars of entitlement. The individual's entitlement period is reduced at a rate in the proportion that the payment is to the monthly assistance allowance to which the individual would have been entitled.

The same payments and conditions are available for tutorial assistance and testing as those under the Post-Vietnam Era GI Bill. Individuals may also receive the actual fee for an admissions or course credit test.[38]

There are four ways in which certain individuals are eligible for an increased allowance:

- Individuals who were eligible for the Post-Korean Conflict GI Bill receive an increase to the monthly allowance, depending on the type of training, rate of pursuit, and number of dependents, for as many months as the individual has remaining Post-Korean Conflict GI Bill entitlement. For example, effective October 1, 2009, an individual in full-time institutional training with two dependents may receive $1,623 monthly.
- Each military branch may provide a College Fund/Kicker at recruitment, which increases the monthly allowance by up to $950 for individuals with critical skills (currently, the Army and Navy provide Kickers to select recruits).

- The military branches may also provide supplemental educational assistance for additional service to active duty service members after they serve an additional five consecutive years on active duty after completing the initial two- or three- year eligibility period of active duty service. Reservists may receive the supplemental educational assistance for additional service after they serve an additional two consecutive years on active duty and four consecutive years in the Selected Reserves, in addition to the initial two-year active duty and four-year Selected Reserves eligibility period.[39] The supplemental educational assistance for additional service is $300 monthly for full-time training (reduced for less than full-time training) and up to an additional $300 (for a total maximum additional amount of $600) monthly for individual with critical skills.
- Service members may also contribute up to an additional $600 while on active duty in $20 monthly increments and receive up to an additional $5 monthly for each $20 contributed over the life of their entitlement period under what is known as the $600 Buy Up Program.

While MGIB-AD basic monthly benefit amounts are adjusted annually, no annual adjustments are made to the additional allowance amounts.

The Tuition Assistance "Top-Up" program was established under the Floyd D. Spence National Defense Authorization Act for Fiscal Year 2001 (P.L. 106-398) to promote retention. Through Tuition Assistance programs, military service branches may pay tuition and expenses for the education and training of active duty personnel. Under Tuition Assistance Top-Up, MGIB-AD service members who have served for at least two years on active duty and who are approved for Tuition Assistance benefits may elect to receive MGIB-AD benefits to pay for education and training expenses above the amount paid by their military service branch. Use of the Top-Up benefit results in a reduction of future MGIB-AD benefits.[40]

Transferability to Dependents

Each DOD service branch is authorized to allow eligible individuals to transfer their educational assistance benefits to family members, but only the Army offers such a program. The Air Force offered a pilot program briefly but has discontinued it. The purpose of the programs is to increase retention of highly qualified and experienced service members.

The Army pilot program is only available to service members in MOS eligible for reenlistment bonuses who elect to participate upon reenlisting for four additional years after serving a minimum of six years. Reservists and National Guard members are not eligible. Benefits may be transferred for up to 18 months to a child[41] who will have finished high school or reached 18 years of age, to a spouse, or to some combination of children and spouse. The spouse may begin using the benefit after the service member completes six years of service; the children must wait until the service member has completed ten years of service. The transferred benefit must be used within ten years of the service member's honorable discharge or before the children reach 26 years of age.[42] In 2009, the Army suggested that it may discontinue the pilot program after August 1, 2009.[43]

Montgomery GI Bill—Selected Reserves

The Montgomery GI Bill-Selected Reserves[44] (MGIB-SR), passed under the same legislation as the MGIB-AD, is a Title 10 U.S.C. DOD program administered by the VA.[45] Each service component of the Selected Reserves is authorized to establish an educational assistance program to encourage membership in the Selected Reserves: Army, Navy, Air Force, Marine Corps, and Coast Guard Reserves; Army National Guard; and the Air National Guard. The benefit is an incentive to stay in the Reserves and was established in recognition of the fact that many states offer educational assistance to Reservists.[46]

Eligible Individuals

The MGIB-SR program is available to individuals serving in the Selected Reserves, including the National Guard, who agree to a six-year service obligation. Educational assistance benefits are available to Selected Reservists who enlist, re-enlist, or extend an enlistment for six years after June 30, 1985, and Reserve officers who agree to serve an additional six years above any existing obligation.[47] The Reservists also have to complete the initial period of active duty for training, complete 180 days of service in the Selected Reserves, have a high school diploma or its equivalent, and satisfactorily meet the necessary training requirements of the Selected Reserves. Individuals who fail to satisfactorily meet the training requirements of the Selected Reserves may be ordered to active duty or required to repay some or all of the educational assistance including interest. The service requirement excludes full-time active duty or full-time National Guard duty for the purpose of organizing, administering, recruiting, instructing, or training the reserve components in a position which is included in the end strength.[48]

Benefit Availability and Duration

Since the obligatory service of six years is the same for all Reservists, the duration of benefits under MGIB-SR is the same for all Reservists—36 months (or the equivalent for part-time educational assistance). Reservists in the MGIB-SR can combine benefits with other educational benefit programs administered by the VA to receive up to 48 months of educational benefits, but cannot receive benefits concurrently from two or more programs. In general, no educational benefits can be paid after separation from the Selected Reserves unless the separation is involuntary or the result of a disability.[49]

Eligible Programs of Education, Institutions, and Establishments

The eligible programs of education, educational institutions, and training establishments are the same as under the MGIB-AD.

Benefit Payments

The educational assistance allowance, paid directly to recipients, is lower than that under the MGIB-AD. Unless on active duty, Reservists make a less time consuming commitment to the military, often working full-time jobs. Also, many states offer educational benefits to Reservists. Reservists called to active duty for extended periods may be eligible for increased benefits under the MGIB-AD, Reserve Educational Assistance Program (discussed later), or Post-9/11 GI Bill (discussed later). Maximum monthly benefit amounts may be adjusted at any time by Congress and are adjusted annually according to the consumer price index for all urban consumers (CPI-U). Effective October 1, 2009, Reservists receive up to $333 monthly according to a schedule based on full-time, three-quarter-time, half-time, and less-than-half-time enrollment. Individuals enrolled less-than-half-time who are also eligible for DOD tuition assistance cannot receive MGIB-SR benefits. For an individual in apprentice or on-the-job training, the monthly allowance is 75%, 55%, and 35% of the monthly benefit otherwise payable to that individual for the first six months, second six months, and thereafter, respectively.[50] Individuals pursuing education exclusively by correspondence receive 55% of the institution's established charges for completed courses, and individuals pursuing education consisting exclusively of flight training receive 60% of the institution's established charges for completed courses.[51]

Individuals may receive up to $2,000 for each licensing or certification test.[52] To improve completion rates, tutorial assistance of up to $1,200 is available under the same conditions as those for the Post-Vietnam Era GI Bill and MGIB-AD.

To improve and target recruitment and retention, each military branch is authorized to provide a College Fund/Kicker at recruitment, which increases the monthly allowance by up to $350 for individuals with critical skills, a specialty in which there is a critical shortage, or a specialty for which it is difficult to recruit or, in the case of critical units, retain. For individuals with critical skills who are also eligible for the MGIB-AD as a result of three years of active duty service, each military branch is also authorized to provide up to an additional $350 (for a total maximum additional amount of $700) monthly.

Transferability to Dependents

Each DOD service branch is authorized to allow eligible individuals to transfer their educational assistance benefits to family members, but no branch currently offers such a program. After serving at least six years in the Selected Reserves and agreeing to serve an additional four years or serving the number of years regulated by the service branch, the authorizing language would allow a member of the Selected Reserves to transfer 18-36 months of benefits to a child who will have finished high school or reached 18 years of age, to a spouse, or to some combination of children and spouse.[53] The eligible Selected Reservist could designate the dependent, the number of months of entitlement, and the period during which it may be used, and modify or revoke the designation at any time. Use of the transferred entitlement period would reduce the entitlement period of the dependent and service member. A spouse could begin using the benefit after the service member completes at least six years of service or the length of service required by regulation; the children would have to wait until the service member completes ten years of service or the length of service required by regulation. The transferred benefit would have to be used before the child reaches 26 years of age. The spouse and children could use the benefit for the same purposes as the Reservists and for the completion of a high school diploma or its equivalent.

Reserve Educational Assistance Program

The Reserve Educational Assistance Program (REAP) was enacted by the Ronald W. Reagan National Defense Authorization Act for FY2005 (P.L. 108-375). It is codified in Title 10 U.S.C., Chapter 1 607.[54] Passage of the program was a direct reaction to the increased number and length of calls to active duty of Reservists that occurred as a result of operations in Afghanistan and Iraq. Reservists must serve at least two continuous years on active duty to receive the MGIB-AD, and the benefits under the MGIB-SR are lower than under the MGIB-AD. REAP sought to provide Reservists with benefits proportional to their active duty service and commensurate with the benefits of the regular Armed Forces.

The purpose is to provide educational assistance to reserve components called to active duty in response to a declared call to war or national emergency. REAP, like the MGIB-SR, is a DOD program administered by the VA. Each DOD branch is required to establish and maintain a program. The program is permanently authorized.

Eligible Individuals

Educational assistance benefits are available to Reservists who have served on active duty in support of a contingency operation for at least 90 consecutive days after September 10, 2001.[55] Benefits are also available to Army National Guard or Air National Guard members who have served on full-time National Guard duty under section 502(f) of Title 32 U.S.C. for at least 90 consecutive days after September 10, 2001, when authorized by the President or Secretary of Defense for the purpose of responding to a national emergency declared by the President and supported by federal funds. The 90-day service requirement is waived for individuals released from duty because of an injury, illness, or disease incurred or aggravated in the line of duty.

Benefit Availability and Duration

As in the MGIBs, most individuals are entitled to educational benefits for a period of up to 36 months (or the equivalent in part-time educational assistance), regardless of the active duty eligibility period. Benefits can be combined with other educational benefit programs administered by the VA using different eligibility periods to receive up to 48 months of educational benefits. In general, no educational benefits can be paid after separation from the Ready Reserves.[56] The Ready Reserves are one of the three major reserve components along with the Standby Reserves and Retired Reserves. The Ready Reserves are the primary manpower pool of the Reserves. They will usually be called to active duty before the other components and include the Selected Reserves.[57] However, individuals who complete the 90-day service requirement and who complete their service contract under honorable conditions remain eligible for benefits for 10 years after separation from the Selected Reserves (separation from other reserve types does not qualify). Also, individuals separated from the Ready Reserve because of a disability which was not the result of the individual's own willful misconduct have ten years from becoming eligible for benefits before the benefits expire.

Eligible Programs of Education, Institutions, and Establishments

The eligible programs of education, educational institutions, and training establishments are the same as under the MGIB-AD.

Benefit Payments

The monthly educational allowance for REAP is a percentage of the allowance provided under the MGIB-AD. Reservists who serve on active duty for at least two continuous years or three aggregate years may receive 80% of the maximum MGIB-AD allowance for that type of education or training, and those serving at least one continuous year may receive 60%. Reservists serving at least 90 consecutive days or released from active duty for an injury, illness, or disease incurred or aggravated as a result of active duty service before serving 90 consecutive days may receive 40% of the maximum MGIB-AD allowance for that type of education or training. Effective October 1, 2009, the maximum allowance for at least two continuous or three aggregate years of active duty service under REAP, $1,094.40, is currently lower than the maximum allowance for at least two years but less than three years of active duty service under the MGIBAD, $1,111.[58] Individuals may receive up to $2,000 for each licensing or certification test.[59]

There are two options for eligible individuals to receive additional educational assistance. Each military branch is authorized to provide a College Fund/Kicker of up to $350 monthly. The $600 Buy-Up program (see the discussion under the MGIB-AD) is also available.

Transferability to Dependents

Each service branch is authorized to allow eligible individuals to transfer their educational assistance benefits to family members, but no branch currently offers such a program. After serving at least six years in the Selected Reserves and agreeing to serve an additional four years or serving the number of years regulated by the service branch, the authorizing language would allow a member of the Selected Reserves to transfer 18-36 months of benefits to a child who will have finished high school or reached 18 years of age, to a spouse, or to some combination of children and spouse.[60] The Reservist could designate the dependent, the number of months of entitlement, and the period during which it may be used, and modify or revoke the designation at any time. The transferred entitlement period would be reduced for the dependent and service member. A spouse could begin using the benefit after the service member completes at least six years of service or the length of service required by regulation; the child would have to wait until the service member has completed ten years of service or the length of service required by regulation. The transferred benefit would have to be used before the child reaches 26 years of age. The spouse and children could use the benefit for the same purposes as the Reservist and for the completion of a high school diploma or its equivalent.

Post-9/11 Veterans Educational Assistance Program

REAP was passed largely in response to concerns about the increased length and hardship of active duty service required of Reservists and National Guard members in military operations in Iraq and Afghanistan. There were four main drivers for the Post-9/11 Veterans Educational Assistance Act of 2008 (P.L. 110-252): providing parity of benefits for Reservists and regular Armed Forces, ensuring comprehensive educational benefits, meeting military recruiting goals, and improving military retention through transferability of benefits. There was a desire for Reservists to receive benefits equivalent to members of the regular Armed Forces for equivalent, though often not continuous, active duty service. While it was recognized that veterans and service members would be eligible for other U.S. Department of Education student financial assistance benefits such as Pell Grants and Stafford Loans,[61] DOD educational assistance, and various state, local, and other federal benefits on top of the basic GI Bill benefits. Members of Congress hoped that a higher benefit would ameliorate military recruiting challenges and reduce the higher unemployment rate among veterans compared with non-veterans of the same age group.[62]

There was some discussion about whether increasing the monthly benefit might result in lower retention in the armed forces. Some DOD research suggested that education is not a very important factor in the decision to stay or leave the military, while other evidence suggested that very high benefits would encourage discharge. The ability to transfer benefits to dependents was considered critical to retention. Only about one-third of eligible individuals had used their MGIB benefits, perhaps because the DOD tuition assistance program allows many service members to achieve a college degree prior to release or discharge. The administration was interested in transferability as well, and President Bush advocated for transferability in his State of the Union address.[63]

The Post-9/11 GI Bill is codified under Title 38 U.S.C., Chapter 33. The stated purpose is to reward members of the armed forces for service on active duty since September 11, 2001; maintain a history of offering educational assistance to veterans; respond to the needs of the armed forces when not at peace; demonstrate the high esteem with which military service is held; recognize the difficult challenges involved in readjusting to civilian life after serving; and enhance the educational assistance benefits to those who serve on active duty after September 11, 2001. The program became effective August 1, 2009. The program is permanently authorized.

Eligible Individuals

Under the Post-9/11 GI Bill, veterans and service members of the Army, Navy, Marine Corps, Air Force, and Coast Guard, including the reserve components and commissioned officers of the Public Health Service (PHS) and the National Oceanic Atmospheric Association (NOAA), may be eligible. Individuals must serve an aggregate minimum of 90 days on active duty after September 10, 2001, or individuals must have been discharged or released after a minimum of 30 continuous days after September 10, 2001, for a service-connected disability. Only a call or order to active duty under section 688, 12301(a), 12301(d), 12301(g), 12302, or 12304 of Title 10 U.S.C. may be included in the active duty service eligibility period required of Reservists. Service by National Guard members or Reservists under a call or order to active duty under Title 32, U.S.C. is not eligible. The active duty service period includes service on active duty in entry-level and skill training if the total active duty service period is at least 24 months.[64] The MGIB-AD and REAP require a certain period of *continuous* active duty service for eligibility; the Post-9/11 GI Bill uses *aggregate* active duty service. The active duty service period excludes time assigned to an education or training program similar to those offered to civilians, excludes time spent as a cadet or midshipman at one of the service academies, excludes other active duty service periods required to meet a service academy or Reserve Officer Training Corps (ROTC) obligation, and excludes service that is terminated because of a defective enlistment and induction. Once the active duty service period is met, individuals must continue on active duty or be discharged with an honorable discharge; be released with honorable service and retired, or transferred to the Reserves or temporary disability list; or be discharged or released for a pre-existing medical condition, hardship, or an interfering physical or mental condition.

Individuals who have not used or who retain an entitlement period under the MGIBs, REAP, and Chapter 107 of Title 10 U.S.C. (professional military education) and individuals who withdrew from the MGIB-AD may make an irrevocable election to receive Post-9/11 GI Bill educational assistance benefits. The individual must be otherwise eligible for the Post-9/11 GI Bill. The decision to receive Post-9/11 GI Bill benefits after using some MGIB-AD benefit does not extend the number of months in the entitlement period. Unused contributions made by the individual to be eligible for the MGIB-AD, up to $1,200, will be refunded as an addition to the last Post-9/11 GI Bill monthly housing allowance once the entitlement period is exhausted. If the individual is not eligible for the monthly housing allowance or fails to exhaust the entitlement period, the unused MGIB-AD contribution will not be refunded. Individuals remain eligible for any supplemental assistance and Kickers; however, they lose any contributions to the MGIB-AD $600 Buy-Up program. [65]

Benefit Availability and Duration

The entitlement period is 36 months. One major difference for veterans discharged with a service connected disability is that under the Post-9/11 GI Bill they are eligible for the maximum (100%) benefit over 36 months, whereas the MGIB-AD only provides one month of entitlement for each month of active duty service, but no more than 36 months. Veterans and service members, many of whom will be eligible for more than one program, can combine benefits with other educational benefit programs administered by the U.S. Department of Veterans Affairs (VA) to receive up to 48 months of educational benefits. By law, no educational benefits under the Post-9/11 GI Bill can be paid 15 years or more after discharge or release from active duty.[66]

Eligible Programs of Education, Institutions, and Establishments

The list of eligible educational institutions and training establishments was narrowed from those in the MGIBs and REAP to include only institutions of higher learning (IHL).[67] The eligible programs of education are courses offered by an IHL and licensing and certification tests.

Benefit Payments

Instead of a single allowance for subsistence, tuition and fees, supplies, books, and equipment paid directly to recipients as in the other GI Bills, eight different payments are available under the Post-9/11 GI Bill:

1. *Tuition.* A per credit hour enrolled tuition payment is made directly to the IHL for each academic term in an amount equal to that charged to the veteran or a percentage of the maximum amount of undergraduate in-state tuition charged for the same number of credit hours at the most expensive public institution in the state in which the individual is enrolled, whichever is less. The percentage of the maximum undergraduate tuition is determined by the length of time served on active duty (**Table 2**). There is great variation among the states, ranging from a low of $90 per credit hour in Puerto Rico[68] to a high of $1,471 in Texas for the 2009-2010 academic year.[69]
   As an example, a Post-9/11 GI Bill eligible veteran with 18 months of qualifying active duty service may choose to enroll as an undergraduate in eight credit hours during one semester at Centralia College in Washington. The veteran will receive

70% of the maximum benefit because the veteran has only 18 months of active duty service. The maximum tuition benefit in Washington state is $380 per credit hour for the 2009-2010 academic year. In the 2007-08 academic year, Centralia College charged $74 per credit hour for in-state part-time undergraduate tuition.[70] Assuming the veteran does not receive institutional aid, Centralia College will charge the veteran $592 ($74 per credit hour × 8 credit hours) for tuition, based on rates for the 2007-08 academic year. Assuming the veteran is only eligible for the basic Post-9/11 GI Bill benefits, the veteran could receive the lesser of $2,128 (70% × $380 per credit hour × 8 credit hours) in Post-9/11 GI Bill tuition benefits for the semester or the actual tuition charged ($592). The VA will send $592 to Centralia College on behalf of the veteran for tuition. The VA will not remit more tuition than the veteran was charged by the institution.

2. *Fees*. A fees payment is made directly to the IHL for each academic term in an amount equal to that charged to the veteran or a percentage of the maximum amount of undergraduate fees charged at the most expensive public institution in the state in which the individual is enrolled, whichever is less. The percentage of the maximum undergraduate fees is determined by the length of time served on active duty (**Table 2**). There is great variation among the states, ranging from a low of $245 in Guam to a high of $63,576.50 in Utah[71] for the 2009-20 10 academic year.[72]
3. *Yellow Ribbon Program Payments*. In cases in which an IHL's tuition and fees are not fully covered by the tuition and fees payment benefits, the IHL may voluntarily enter into a Yellow Ribbon Program agreement with the U.S. Department of Veterans Affairs (VA) to match an equal percentage of some portion of the remaining tuition and fees (see "Yellow Ribbon Program" section below).
4. *Housing Allowance*. Individuals who are on active duty, enrolled half-time or less, or in a program offered exclusively through distance learning[73] are not eligible for the Post-9/11 GI Bill housing allowance. Individuals not so excluded may directly receive a percentage of an amount which equals the monthly basic allowance for housing (BAH) for a member of the Armed Forces with dependents in pay grade E-5 in the military housing area in which the IHL is located.[74] The percentage of the monthly housing allowance is determined by the length of time served on active duty (**Table 2**). There is great variation among the localities in the United States, ranging from a low of $801 in the Mansfield, OH, area to a high of $2,751 in the New York City area in 2009.[75]
5. *Books and Supplies Stipend*. Individuals who are not on active duty and individuals who are enrolled more than half-time may also receive a percentage of the annual stipend for books and required educational expenses. The maximum stipend is $1,000 per year. The percentage of the stipend is determined by the length of time served on active duty (**Table 2**). The stipend is paid each term based on the number of credit hours, or their equivalent, in which the individual is enrolled. Each credit hour, or its equivalent, is worth $41.67.[76] This stipend does not reduce the entitlement period and does not reduce other benefit payments.
6. *Tutorial Assistance*. An individual is entitled to payment, not to exceed $100 monthly and up to a maximum of $1,200 over the course of the entitlement period, for tutorial assistance provided it is certified by the IHL that the individual needs tutoring to pass a course required for the approved program of education. The

maximum tutorial assistance is not reduced depending on the length of active duty service. Tutorial assistance is available in the MGIBs and REAP; however, the tutorial assistance in the Post-9/11 GI Bill does not reduce the entitlement period and does not reduce other benefit payments.

7. *Testing and Certification Fees*. A fee of up to $2,000 for one approved licensing or certification test may be paid to an individual regardless of whether the individual passes the test. The maximum fee is not reduced depending on the length of active duty service. Licensing and certification test fees are available under the MGIBs and REAP; however, the fee does not reduce the entitlement period and does not reduce other benefit payments under the Post-9/11 GI Bill. The REAP and MGIBs place no limit on the number of tests for which an allowance may be paid as long as each payment for each test does not exceed $2,000.
8. *Relocation and Travel Assistance*. An individual who resides in a rural county and who has to relocate a distance of at least 500 miles, or an individual who must travel by air to attend an IHL, is entitled to a single payment of up to $500. The relocation assistance does not reduce the entitlement period, does not reduce other benefit payments, and is not reduced depending on the length of active duty service.

Payments for individuals who are on active duty or enrolled half-time or less are slightly different. Individuals on active duty may only receive (payable to the IHL) for each academic term the amount of tuition and fees charged by the IHL, but the amount cannot duplicate any amounts received through a DOD Tuition Assistance Program.[77] This amount could exceed the amounts charged by most expensive public institution in the state. Individuals on active duty may not receive the housing allowance or books and supplies stipend. Individuals enrolled half-time or less may only receive (payable to the IHL) for each academic term the amount charged by the IHL, but not more than the amount the individual would have been eligible to receive if enrolled full-time.[78] Individuals enrolled half-time or less may not receive the housing allowance, but they may receive a books and supplies stipend reduced in proportion to the attendance rate. Individuals on active duty and those enrolled half-time or less may still be eligible to receive tutorial assistance, testing and certification fees, and relocation and travel assistance.

Individuals may be eligible for advance payments, supplemental assistance for additional years of service, Kickers, and Tuition Assistance Top-Up. Individuals who pursue all courses online are not eligible for Kickers because Kickers are added to the monthly housing allowance, which they do not receive. Individuals who enroll half-time or less or who are serving on active duty are also not eligible for Kickers.[79] Advance payment of the housing allowance (payable to the IHL) is available to individuals enrolled more than half-time, but tuition, fees, and books and supplies costs cannot be advanced. [80] The supplemental assistance for additional years of service and Kickers may be reduced depending on the individual's time served on active duty. Individuals in the Post-9/11 GI Bill forfeit any contributions to the $600 Buy Up program.

Yellow Ribbon Program

The Yellow Ribbon G.I. Education Enhancement Program covers a portion of the tuition and fees that exceed the base Post-9/11 GI Bill benefit. The Yellow Ribbon Program payment is paid equally by the IHL and the VA. The program allows IHLs to enter into agreements with the VA to match a certain amount of the tuition and fees not already covered by the basic Post-9/11 GI Bill.[81] Each IHL must establish the number of eligible individuals it is willing to support and how much it is willing to contribute for each individual. VA regulations allow IHLs to specify their support by each sub-element: college or professional school; and by student status: undergraduate, graduate, or doctoral.[82] The program is only available to individuals who have served on active duty for 36 months and those who were discharged due to a service-connected disability after 30 consecutive days of active duty service. As long as the IHL remains in the Yellow Ribbon Program, an individual admitted under the program who maintains satisfactory progress will continue to be supported under the program. As of June 24, 2009, the VA had entered into over 2,500 Yellow Ribbon agreements with about 700 public and private schools in all 50 states, the District of Columbia, and Puerto Rico. The schools have agreed to support between one and an unlimited number of eligible students for $50 per semester to the maximum amount needed by the student.

For example, a Post-9/11 GI Bill eligible veteran with 36 months of qualifying active duty service may choose to enroll as a graduate student in eight credit hours during one semester at Gonzaga University in Washington. The base Post-9/11 GI Bill benefit covers the maximum amount of *undergraduate* tuition charged at a public institution in the state. The veteran will receive 100% of the maximum benefit because the veteran has 36 months of active duty service. In the 2007-08 academic year, Gonzaga University charged $670 per credit hour for part-time graduate tuition and $176 per year in full-time graduate student fees.[83] For the 2009-2010 academic year, the maximum charge per credit hour at the most expensive public institution in Washington is $380, and the maximum fees for an academic term at the most expensive public institution in the state are $14,444.50. Assuming the veteran does not receive institutional aid, Gonzaga University will charge the veteran a total of $5,448, composed of $5,360 ($670 per credit hour × 8 credit hours) in tuition and $88 ($176 fees per year × 1/2 for one semester) in fees. Assuming the veteran is only eligible for the basic Post-9/11 GI Bill benefits, the veteran could receive the lesser of $3,040 (100% × $380 per credit hour × 8 credit hours) in Post-9/11 GI Bill tuition benefits for the semester or the actual tuition charged ($5,360), and the lesser of $14,444.50 in Post-9/11 GI Bill fees benefits for the semester or the actual fees charged ($88). For the basic Post-9/11 GI Bill benefits, the VA will send $3,040 to the University on behalf of the veteran for tuition. For the basic Post-9/11 GI Bill benefits, the VA will send $88 to the university on behalf of the veteran for fees. In summary, the veteran has been charged $5,448 in tuition and fees, and the VA has paid $3,128 ($3,040 tuition + $88 fees) in basic benefits, leaving an unpaid balance of $2,320 ($5,448 - $3,128). Under the Yellow Ribbon Program in 2009-2010, Gonzaga University has agreed to support 25 students for up to $11,420 per student per year. If the veteran in this example is one of the 25 students, the VA will match the university's payment up to $11,420 per year or $5,710 per semester. Therefore, the VA will make a Yellow Ribbon payment of $1,160, the lesser of half of the unpaid balance $1,160 ($2,320 ÷ 2) or $5,710. The VA will have paid $4,288 ($3,128 in basic tuition and fees + $1,160 in Yellow Ribbon payments) on behalf of the veteran. The Post-9/11 GI Bill will provide the veteran a total of $5,448 ($4,288 from the VA + $1,160 from the university) for tuition and fees. The veteran will not need to provide any additional out-of-pocket funds for tuition and fees charges.

Table 2. Percentage of Maximum Post-9/11 GI Bill Benefits based on Aggregate Length of Active Duty Service

Aggregate time served on active duty since 9/11/2001	Percentage of maximum benefit payable
At least 36 months	100
At least 30 continuous days on active duty and discharged due to service- connected disability	100
At least 30 months, but less than 36 months	90
At least 24 months, but less than 30 months	80
At least 18 months, but less than 24 months	70
At least 12 months, but less than 18 months	60
At least 6 months, but less than 12 months	50
At least 90 days, but less than 6 months	40

Source: Prepared by CRS based on Title 38 U.S.C. § 3313 and data available from the U.S. Department of Veterans Affairs.

Marine Gunnery Sergeant John David Fry Scholarship Program

The Supplemental Appropriations Act of 2009 (P.L. 111-32) amended the Post-9/11 GI Bill to create the Marine Gunnery Sergeant John David Fry Scholarship. The scholarship program is available to the children of individuals who, on or after September 11, 2001, die in the line of duty while serving on active duty as a member of the Armed Forces. The definition of children is the same as it is in the MGIB-AD, but also includes married children and children over 23 years of age.[84] The Armed Forces include the Reserves and National Guard. Scholarship recipients are eligible to receive all Post-9/11 GI Bill benefits for 36 months at the maximum 100% rate. No scholarship program benefits can be paid 15 years or more after the child's 18th birthday. Although the program took effect August 1, 2009, payments, including retroactive payments, will not be made until August 1, 2010.

The VA has established rules for individuals who are eligible for the scholarship and who have served in the Armed Forces. Children who are eligible under the MGIBs or REAP must relinquish eligibility under one of those programs to receive benefits under the Post-9/11 GI Bill. Children who are serving on active duty will receive benefits like other service members on active duty.[85]

Transferability to Dependents

The DOD allows the transfer of benefits from individuals eligible for the Post-9/11 GI Bill to certain family members.[86] The Post-9/11 GI Bill-eligible individual must be a member of the Armed Forces (active duty or Selected Reserves) on or after August 1, 2009. Three categories of individuals may transfer some or all of their benefits. The first category includes service members who have completed six years of service and agree to serve four additional years. The second category includes service members who have completed ten years of service and are precluded from serving an additional four years but agree to serve the maximum amount of time allowable. The third category includes service members who become retirement eligible between August 1, 2009, and August 1, 2013. Service members in the third category are required to serve an additional 0-3 years, depending on their retirement eligibility date.[87]

Individuals eligible to transfer their benefits can transfer up to 36 months of benefits to their child, to their spouse, or to some combination of children and spouse.[88] The family members must be enrolled in the DOD Defense Eligibility Enrollment Reporting System and be eligible for benefits at the time the transfer is designated. The eligible service member can designate the family member, the number of months of the entitlement period, and the period during which it may be used, and can modify or revoke the designation at any time. After retirement or separation from the Armed Forces, the individual can only modify the number of months of the transferred entitlement period or revoke the designation for those family members who have received transferred benefits before the retirement or separation. After retirement or separation from the Armed Forces, the individual cannot add new family members. As the dependent uses the transferred benefit, the remaining entitlement periods of both the dependent and service member are reduced. The designees can use the benefit for the same purposes as the eligible individual and for the completion of a high school diploma or its equivalent.

A spouse can begin using the benefit after the service member completes at least six years of service or the length of service required by regulation. A spouse who subsequently divorces the Post-9/11 GI Bill-eligible individual is still eligible to use the transferred benefits unless the eligible individual revokes the transfer. The spouse receives payments according to the current status of the eligible individual. The spouse may use the benefit within 15 years of the eligible individual's discharge or release from active duty service.

Children have to achieve a high school diploma or its equivalent or reach 18 years of age before using the benefit. The service member has to complete at least ten years of service or the length of service required by regulation before the designated children can use the benefit. Children receive payments as if the eligible individual were not on active duty. Children must use the benefit before reaching 26 years of age.

Survivors' and Dependents' Educational Assistance Program

The Survivors' and Dependents' Educational Assistance Program (DEA) was first established by the War Orphans' Educational Assistance Act of 1956 (P.L. 84-634). The DEA program is codified under Title 38 U.S.C., Chapter 35. The benefit allows eligible individuals to attain the education they would have or maintain the standard of living they would have if the service member had not become disabled, delayed,[89] or died as a result of military service.

Eligible Individuals

Educational assistance benefits are available to

- the child or spouse of a person who died of a service-connected disability resulting from active duty service, has a total permanent disability[90] as a result of an active duty service-connected disability, or died while the active duty service- connected disability was being evaluated;[91]
- the child or spouse of a person who has been listed as missing in action, captured in the line of duty, or forcibly detained as a result of active duty service; and

- the spouse or child of a person who is hospitalized or receiving outpatient medical care, services, or treatment as a result of a total permanent disability incurred in or aggravated by active duty service and who is likely to be discharged or released as a result of the disability.

The military service of the person who was disabled, delayed, or died must not have terminated under dishonorable conditions. The definition of children is the same as it is in the MGIB-AD, but also includes married children and children over 23 years of age.[92] Neither the spouse nor child may receive educational assistance under DEA while in the armed forces or if released under dishonorable conditions.

Benefit Availability and Duration

Educational benefits may be paid to the spouse for ten years from the date of death of the veteran or from the date of VA notification of eligibility due to the veteran's condition.[93] If the service member dies on active duty, or total permanent disability as a result of a service-connected disability is determined within three years of discharge, the spouse may use the benefits for 20 years. Educational benefits may be paid to children after they achieve a high school diploma or its equivalent, or after they reach 18 years of age, but before they reach 26 years of age.[94] Individuals are entitled to 45 months (or the equivalent in part-time attendance) of educational and training benefits.

Eligible Programs of Education, Institutions, and Establishments

The list of eligible educational institutions are the same as under VEAP. The eligible training establishments are establishments providing apprentice or other on-the-job training. The eligible programs of education are courses at an educational institution that lead to the attainment of a predetermined educational, vocational, or professional objective; and preparatory course(s) for IHE and graduate school admissions. Eligible programs also include licensing or certification tests for a predetermined vocation or profession, provided such tests and the licensing or credentialing organizations or entities that offer such tests are approved; national tests for admission to institutions of higher learning or graduate schools (such as the Scholastic Aptitude Test (SAT)); and national tests providing an opportunity for course credit at an IHL (such as an Advanced Placement (AP) exam). Secondary education for those without a high school diploma or its equivalent, secondary education in preparation for postsecondary education, specialized vocational courses required because of a mental or physical handicap, and special restorative training[95] are also eligible programs of education.

Benefit Payments

An allowance for subsistence, tuition and fees, supplies, books, and equipment is paid directly to recipients. Maximum monthly benefit amounts may be adjusted at any time by Congress and are adjusted annually according to the consumer price index (all items, U. S. city average). Effective October 1, 2009, individuals receive up to $925 monthly according to a schedule based on full-time, three-quarter-time, and half-time institutional enrollment and $925 monthly for cooperative training. Individuals enrolled less than half-time but more than quarter-time at an institution receive the lesser of actual tuition and fees or $461 monthly, and individuals enrolled quarter-time or less receive the lesser of actual tuition and fees or

$231.25 monthly. Individuals receive up to $745 monthly according to a schedule based on full-time, three-quarter-time, and half-time farm cooperative training. Only spouses may pursue education exclusively by correspondence and receive 55% of the institution's established charges for completed courses.[96] For individuals in apprentice or on-the-job training, the monthly allowance is $674, $505, $333, and $168 for the first six months, second six months, third six months, and thereafter, respectively.[97] Tutorial assistance of up to $1,200 is available under the same conditions as those for the Post-Vietnam Era GI Bill. Individuals may receive up to $2,000 for a licensing or certification test, and individuals may receive the actual fee for an admissions or course credit test.[98]

The DEA Program provides two categories of assistance to disadvantaged individuals:

- Special assistance to the educationally disadvantaged allows individuals who do not have a high school diploma or its equivalent and who are in need of some secondary school preparation in order to pursue a postsecondary education to receive a monthly educational assistance allowance. Benefits do not reduce the basic entitlement period for the first five months. Individuals pursuing a high school diploma may receive the lesser of actual tuition and fees or the full-time institutional monthly rate.
- The second category of assistance is special restorative training to overcome, or reduce, the effects of a manifest physical or mental disability which would handicap a person (other than the spouse of a person delayed) in the pursuit of a program of education. The entitlement period may be extended beyond 45 months to accomplish the special restorative training. Individuals receive $925 monthly for full-time[99] special restorative training and an increased amount equal to the amount that the tuition and fees for the training exceeds $287 monthly.[100]

For those children and spouses who may also be eligible for pension, compensation, or dependency and indemnity compensation, the legislation bars some recipients from accepting DEA educational assistance and pension, compensation, or dependency and indemnity compensation. A spouse, a child under 18 years of age, and a helpless child may receive DEA educational assistance and pension, compensation, or dependency and indemnity compensation concurrently. Once a child over 18 years of age begins receiving DEA educational assistance, the child can no longer receive payment or increased rates, or additional amounts of pension, compensation, or dependency and indemnity compensation based on school attendance.[101]

Summary and Comparison of Programs

VEAP, MGIB-AD, MGIB-SR, REAP, and the Post-9/11 GI Bill programs are available as of August 1, 2009. Many service members are eligible for more than one program. The programs, with the exception of the Post-9/11 GI Bill, provide assistance for the same programs of education at very different payment rates. There are also variations in the length of time during which the benefits must be used. Despite the fact that the VA expects most veterans and service members to choose the Post-9/11 GI Bill, all new recruits to the regular Armed Forces will contribute to the MGIB-AD unless they decline the benefit. Eligible individuals will need a significant understanding of the programs in order to determine which program will be the most advantageous to their situation.

Transferability of Benefits between Programs

Veterans and service members, many of whom will be eligible for more than one program, can combine benefit programs administered by the VA to receive up to 48 months of educational benefits; however, benefits under more than one program cannot be received concurrently.[102] An individual may receive credit for service under only one program and must elect the program to which such service is to be credited. This decision is generally irrevocable. The decision regarding from which program to receive benefits may be changed once each calendar month except for changes to or from the Post-9/11 GI Bill, which can only be changed once each academic term.

Reserves and National Guard Eligibility

Program eligibility for Reservists and National Guard members is variable across the programs. Reservists who made contributions to their educational fund while on active duty, excluding active duty for training, for at least 180 days are eligible for VEAP. Three groups are eligible under the MGIB-AD:

- Selected Reservists and National Guard members who serve two continuous years of honorable active duty service under Title 10 U.S.C. § 12103(d);
- individuals serving on certain full-time National Guard duty for the purpose of organizing, administering, recruiting, instructing, or training the National Guard under Title 32 U.S.C.; and
- a small group of National Guard members who first served on full-time National Guard active duty under Title 32 U.S.C. between June 30, 1985, and November 29, 1989, and who made the requisite $1,200 contribution during the open period from October 9, 1996, to June 8, 1997.

The MGIB-SR does not require any active duty service. All members of the Selected Reserves, including National Guard, are eligible if they agree to a six-year service obligation.

Two groups are eligible under REAP:

- Reservists, including National Guard, who have served on active duty in support of a contingency operation for at least 90 consecutive days after September 10, 2001; and
- National Guard members who have served on full time National Guard duty under Title 32 U.S.C. § 502(f) for at least 90 consecutive days after September 10, 2001, when authorized by the President or Secretary of Defense for the purpose of responding to a national emergency declared by the President and supported by federal funds.

Table 3. Selected Characteristics of Veterans' Educational Assistance Programs

Characteristic	VEAP	MGIB-AD	MGIB-SR	REAP	Post-9/11 GI Bill	DEA
Year enacted	1976	1984	1984	2004	2008	1956
Initial authorization	P.L. 94-502	P.L. 98-525	P.L. 98-525	P.L. 108-375	P.L. 110-252	P.L. 84-634
Eligible Individuals						
Period of qualifying service	12/31/1976 to 7/1/1985	Entered active duty after 6/30/1985	7/1/1985 to present	After 9/10/2001 to present	After 9/10/2001 to present	After the beginning of the Spanish American War
Minimum required length of service	181 continuous days of active duty service, if entered before October 16, 1981 24 months of continuous active duty service if entered after October 16, 1981	181 continuous days of active duty service; 24 months of active duty if enlisted after September 7, 1980	Accepted 6-year reserve obligation after June 30, 1985	90 days of consecutive service in a contingency operation	90 aggregate days of active duty service	None
Discharge status	Other than dishonorable or on active duty	Fully honorable discharge or on active duty	Must remain with Reserve unit	Honorable separation or further service in Reserves	Honorable discharge or further service in Reserves	Other than dishonorable or on active duty
Contribution	$25 to $100 per month; $2,700 maximum	Pay reduction of $100 per month for the first 12 months of pay	None	None	None	None

Table 3. (Continued)

Characteristic	VEAP	MGIB-AD	MGIB-SR	REAP	Post-9/11 GI Bill	DEA
Benefit Availability and Duration						
Period of use	1/1/1977 to present	7/1/1985 to present	7/1/1985 to present	12/9/2001 to present	Starting 8/1/2009	1956 to present
Duration of benefits	Lesser of 36 months or number of months of contributions	Lesser of 36 months or number of months of active duty and onequarter number of months of Reserve duty	36 months	36 months	36 months	45 months
General time limitation on use of benefits	Within 10 years of discharge or release from active duty	Within 10 years of discharge or release from active duty or required Reserve duty	While in the Selected Reserves	While in the Ready Reserves Within 10 years of Selected Rese-rves separation Within 10 years of Ready Reserves separa-tion due to Certain disabilities	Within 15 years of discharge or release from active duty	For the spouse: within 10 years of eligibility, or within 20 in some instantces For the child: after finishing high school or reaching age 18, but before reaching age 26
Eligible Programs of Education, Institutions, and Establishments						
Institution of higher learning	Eligible	Eligible	Eligible	Eligible	Eligible	Eligible
Apprentice and on-the-job training	Eligible	Eligible	Eligible	Eligible	Not eligible	Eligible
Entrepreneurship training	Eligible	Eligible	Eligible	Eligible	Not eligible	Eligible

Table 3. (Continued)

Characteristic	VEAP	MGIB-AD	MGIB-SR	REAP	Post-9/11 GI Bill	DEA
Cooperative training	Eligible	Eligible	Eligible	Eligible	Not eligible	Eligible
Licensing and certification tests	Eligible	Eligible	Eligible	Eligible	Eligible	Eligible
Admissions or course credit tests	Eligible	Eligible	Eligible	Eligible	Not eligible	Eligible
Tutorial assistance	Eligible	Eligible	Eligible	Eligible	Eligible	Not eligible
Benefit Payments						
Maximum standard benefit as of October 1, 2008	$300 per month[a] for subsistence, tuition and fees, supplies, books, and equipment	$1,321 per monthb for subsistence, tuition and fees, supplies, books, and equipment	$329 per month[b] for subsistence, tuition and fees, supplies, books, and equipment	$1,057 per month[c] for subsistence, tuition and fees, supplies, books, and equipment	$2,751 per month for subsistence[d] Up to $1,471 tuition per credit hour per academic term[d] Up to $63,576.50 for fees per academic term[d]	$915 per month for subsistence, tuition and fees, supplies, books, and equipment
Books and supplies	Not eligible	Not eligible	Not eligible	Not eligible	Up to $1,000 annually	Not eligible
Relocation allowance	Not eligible	Not eligible	Not eligible	Not eligible	Up to $500 once	Not eligible
Maximum tutorial assistance	$1,200	$1,200	$1,200	$1,200	$1,200	$1,200
Maximum licensing and certification test fees	$2,000 per test	$2,000 per test	$2,000 per test	$2,000 per test	$2,000 for one test	$2,000 per test

Table 3. (Continued)

Characteristic	VEAP	MGIB-AD	MGIB-SR	REAP	Post-9/11 GI Bill	DEA
Admissions or course credit test	Actual cost	Actual cost	Eligible	Eligible	Not eligible	Eligible
Advance payments	Eligible	Eligible	Eligible	Eligible	Eligible	Eligible
Accelerated payments	Not eligible	Eligible	Eligible	Eligible	Not eligible	Not eligible
Tuition Assist-ance Top Up Program	Not eligible	Eligible	Not eligible	Not eligible	Eligible	Not eligible
$600 Buy Up Program	Not eligible	Eligible	Eligible	Eligible	Not eligible	Not eligible
College Fund/Kicker	Not eligible	Eligible	Eligible	Eligible	Eligible	Not eligible
		Up to $950 per month for recur-itment Up to $350 per month for retention	Up to $350 per month	Up to $350 per month	Up to $950 per month[e] for Recruitment Up to $350 per month for retention	
Supplemental assistance for critical skills	Not eligible	Up to $300 per month	Up to $300 per month	Not eligible	Up to $300 per month	Not eligible
Supplemental educational assistance for additional service	Not eligible	$300 per month	Not eligible	Not eligible	Up to $300 per month	Not eligible

Table 3. (Continued)

Characteristic	VEAP	MGIB-AD	MGIB-SR	REAP	Post-9/11 GI Bill	DEA
Transferability to dependents						
Transferability to dependents	Not authorized	Authorized. Army pilot program available	Authorized	Authorized	Authorized. DOD Policy issued 6/23/2009 Scholarship program for children of deceased	Not authorized

Source: Prepared by CRS based on data available from the VA; Title 38 U.S.C., Chapters 30 and 33; and Title 10 U.S.C., Chapters 1606 and 1607.

a. Government matches every $1 the service member contributes with $2. The maximum benefit available under the program is $8,100 ($5,400 federal contribution and $2,700 individual contribution). The total contribution (service member contribution plus government share) is than divided by the number of months the service member contributed to VEAP.

b. Amounts shown are for full-time institutional training, and for individuals who completed a minimum of three years of service. The amounts are less for individuals who served less than three years and who attend less than full-time. The educational benefits payment rate schedule is available at http://www.gibill.va.gov/GI_Bill_Info/rates.htm. The MGIB-AD maximum payment does not reflect the allowance received by Post-Korean Conflict GI Bill recipients who transfer to the program.

c. The monthly amount is a percentage of the MGIB-AD and is based on the number of continuous days of active duty service. The amount shown is for full-time institutional training, and for individuals who completed at least two years of active duty service. The amount is less for individuals who served two years or less, and who attend less than full-time.

d. The maximum standard benefit varies depending on the location of the IHL. The maximum standard tuition and fees depend on the state in which the IHL resides and are based upon the 2009-2010 academic year, while the maximum standard housing allowance depends on the locale in which the IHL resides.

e. Individuals eligible for MGIB-SR who elect to receive benefits under the Post-9/11 GI Bill may be eligible to receive up to $350 per month from the college fund/kicker.

Reservists, including National Guard, who are called or ordered to active duty under section 688, 12301(a), 12301(d), 12301(g), 12302, or 12304 of Title 10 U.S.C. for an aggregate minimum of 90 days after September 10, 2001, are eligible for the Post-9/11 GI Bill.

Permanent Authorization of Programs

As currently enacted, the MGIBs, REAP, Post-9/11, and DEA programs will persist indefinitely because the periods of eligibility are unrestricted into the future, and Congress has not specified an end date after which no benefits would be paid. VEAP participation may slowly end, as service members on active duty between January 1, 1977, and June 30, 1985, are less likely to pursue education and more likely to transfer the remaining entitlement to benefits to one of the newer programs.

Veterans Counseling

For the most part, individuals receiving educational assistance under the VEAP, MGIBs, REAP, Post-9/11 GI Bill, or DEA may request counseling from the VA. The counseling may include, but is not limited to, assistance selecting a program of education, resolving personal problems, and resolving academic difficulties. Counseling was provided to all recipients of educational assistance until 1972. Counseling is still required under DEA for a child who may require specialized vocational training or special restorative training, or a child who is under 18 years of age and has not completed high school. It is also required for a spouse who desires specialized vocational training. Counseling is still required under all of the programs if the individual is rated as incompetent.

Comparison of Educational Assistance Programs

Table 3 provides a summary of some of the key characteristics of the active programs.

The active duty eligibility requirements between the three main programs that offer benefits for active duty service (MGIB-SR does not offer benefits for active duty service and VEAP participation is low) create some differences in benefits (see **Table 4**). Comparing benefits is complicated by the fact that MGIB-AD and REAP only take into account consecutive or continuous periods of service; while the Post-9/11 GI Bill computes aggregate periods of service. Also, estimating payments under the Post-9/11 GI Bill is complicated by the fact that some of the published maximum fees for each state are inflated by small programs at a small number of institutions in the state. For instance, the Post-9/11 GI Bill 200 8-2009 maximum total fees per term for Colorado are $43,035, but the maximum in-state required fees for most full-time undergraduates in the 28 public two- and four-year IHEs in the state of Colorado is $1,379 for the full 2007-2008 academic year.[103] Students who attended the helicopter pilot training program at Aims Community College in Colorado were charged $43,035 in fees per term during the 2008- 2009 academic year.[104]

Table 4. Annual payments for the MGIB-AD, REAP, and Post-9/11 GI Bill based on Length of Active Duty Service Requirement Full-Time Enrollment at an IHL for Nine Months

Active duty service requirement	MGIB-AD maximum standard annual payment ($)[ab]		REAP maximum standard annual payment ($)[a]	Post-9/11 GI Bill estimated median annual payment ($)[ac]
	Reservists	Regular		
90 days	—	—	4,756	12,936
6 months	—	—	4,756	16,170
12 months	—	—	7,133	19,404
18 months	—	—	7,133	22,638
2 years[d]	9,657	9,657	9,511	25,872
2 ½ years[d]	9,657	9,657	9,511	29,107
3 years	11,889	11,889	9,511	32,341

Source: Prepared by CRS based on Title 38 U.S.C., Chapters 30 and 33; Title 10 U.S.C., Chapter 1607; and data available from the VA.

a. The annual payments exclude additional allowances for tutorial assistance, licensing and certification fees, kickers, the $600 Buy-Up Program, additional assistance for additional service, and additional payments for critical skills.

b. The MGIB-AD maximum standard annual payment does not reflect the allowance received by Post-Korean Conflict GI Bill recipients who transfer to the program.

c. The Post-9/11 GI Bill estimated median annual payment is the un-weighted median annual payment of all 50- state basic allowance for housing (BAH) areas. The annual payment was calculated to estimate full-time IHL attendance for an academic year by a veteran by summing for each BAH within a state the 2009 monthly housing allowance times nine months, the 2008-2009 maximum charge per credit hour for the state times 24 credit hours, and the 2008-2009 maximum total fees per term times two terms. The estimated median annual payment is the average of the two values in the middle of the distribution—the Rockford, IL, area with a BAH of $965, maximum charge per credit hour of $558.08, and maximum total fees per term of $5,126.50 and the Ocala, FL, area with a BAH of $1,070, maximum charge per credit hour of $682.23, and maximum total fees per term of $3,172.86. Using this methodology, benefit recipients in the Denver, CO, area with a BAH of $1,531, maximum charge per credit hour of $419, and maximum total fees per term of $43,035 could receive the highest estimated annual payment of up to $109,905. Benefit recipients in the Fort Chaffee/Fort Smith, AR, area with a BAH of $776, maximum charge per credit hour of $167, and maximum total fees per term of $751.46 could receive the lowest estimated annual payment of up to $12,494.92. The estimate does not include possible participation in the Yellow Ribbon Program, a books and supplies stipend, and relocation and travel assistance.

d. Reservists must fulfill an additional four years of Reserve duty in addition to the active duty requirements to receive the MGIB-AD payment.

For an eligible Reservists who has 90 consecutive days of active duty service and attends an IHL full-time for nine months, the estimated median annual benefit under the Post-9/11 GI Bill ($12,936) is almost triple the benefit under REAP ($4,756). A member of the regular armed forces who serves two continuous years on active duty may be eligible to receive double the benefit under the Post-9/11 GI Bill ($19,629) compared to MGIB-AD ($9,657). A Reservist who serves two continuous years on active duty may be eligible to receive an estimated median annual benefit of $25,872 under the Post-9/11 GI Bill without the MGIB-

AD requirement of an additional four years in the Selected Reserves in order to be eligible to receive a maximum standard annual MGIB-AD benefit of $9,657.

RELATED DEPARTMENT OF VETERANS AFFAIRS PROGRAMS

Vocational Rehabilitation and Employment Program

The Vocational Rehabilitation and Employment Program (VR&E) is discussed as a related program because veterans who are eligible for both the MGIB-AD and VR&E must choose which program they want to receive educational benefits under. In 1918, Congress passed the Vocational Rehabilitation Act (P.L. 65-178) to provide maximum independence and the retraining and placing in productive occupations of disabled persons who had served in the U.S. military and naval forces.[105] Under the current program, eligible veterans must have served on active duty after September 16, 1940, and been discharged under circumstances other than dishonorable. Also, eligible veterans must have a service-connected disability employment handicap rating of at least 20% or a serious employment handicap rating of 10% as a result of a disability incurred in or aggravated by service for which a pension is payable under the laws administered by the VA, or would be but for the receipt of retirement pay. In addition, eligible veterans must be in need of vocational rehabilitation to overcome the handicap caused by the service-connected disability. Veterans are entitled to the program within 12 years of discharge or release.

Veterans receiving VR&E services receive counseling to provide an initial evaluation, develop a plan for rehabilitation or employment, and overcome any problems that arise during the implementation of the plan for rehabilitation or employment. The counseling may be psychological, vocational, personal adjustment, employment, or educational.

After evaluation of the veterans' condition and development of an individualized rehabilitation plan, eligible veterans will be assigned to either a vocational rehabilitation program or a program of independent living services and assistance. If it is determined that the achievement of a vocational goal is feasible, the individual will be assigned to a vocational rehabilitation program, which may include counseling, diagnostic, medical, social, psychological, independent living, economic, educational, vocational, and employment services. Eligible programs of education are the same as under the VEAP.

With some exceptions, the program provides 48 months to accomplish the individualized vocational rehabilitation plan.[106] While pursuing the plan, the individual's progress is tracked and reviewed by a case manager to ensure the veteran has all the necessary resources to be successful. Eligible veterans receive a subsistence allowance based on the number of dependents, type of education or training pursued, and rate of attendance. Effective October 1, 2009, the allowance for full-time training at an IHL is $800.36 monthly for an individual with two dependents. Individuals who pursue non-pay or nominal pay on-the-job training in a federal, state, local, or federally recognized Indian tribe agency; training in the home; vocational coursework in a rehabilitation facility or sheltered workshop; or institutional non-farm cooperative training lessthan-full-time are not eligible to receive the monthly subsistence allowance. Veterans may receive advance payments and may receive the subsistence allowance during authorized leaves of absence. The case manager may authorize equipment, supplies, and incidental goods and services to ensure the veteran's success as long as the cost of the incidental goods and services does not exceed 5% of the annual training cost. After successful completion of the individualized rehabilitation plan, veterans may be eligible to receive two additional months of the subsistence allowance while receiving employment placement services.

Veterans eligible for and entitled to the MGIB-AD may choose to receive the subsistence allowance and other benefits available under the MGIB-AD while pursuing the individualized rehabilitation plan, but they forfeit access to the VR&E subsistence allowance, loans, tutorial assistance, tuition, fees, books, supplies, handling charges, licensing fees, equipment, and other training materials. While receiving an allowance under the MGIB-AD, the veteran must abide by all of the provisions of the MGIB-AD program. The law does not provide for similar coordination of benefits between the VR&E and Post-9/11 GI Bill programs.

Veterans who are also eligible to receive the disability compensation[107] as a result of hospital treatment or observation may not receive the total VR&E or MGIB-AD allowance and disability compensation in excess of the greater of 100% disability compensation or the sum of the VR&E or MGIB-AD allowance and the amount of disability compensation that would be paid to the veteran if he or she was not receiving compensation at such a rate as the result of that hospital treatment or observation.

Veterans Work-Study

The Veterans Work Study Program is discussed as a related program because it allows VEAP, MGIB-AD, MGIB-SR, and Post-9/11 GI Bill participants to receive additional financial assistance through the VA. The program is codified in Title 38 U.S.C. § 3485. Veterans and Reservists in the VEAP, MGIBs, Post-9/11 GI Bill, and VR&E who are enrolled at least threequarter-time may take advantage of a VA administered work-study program. Individuals in the DEA who are enrolled at least three-quarter-time in the United States and are not pursuing a program of special restorative training may also take advantage of a VA administered work-study program. Although veterans with at least a 30% disability rating[108] receive priority in the selection of program participants, the VA also considers the individual's need for additional educational assistance, whether the individual has the necessary access to transportation to and from the work site, the individual's motivation, and the individual's compatibility with the available work assignments.

An individual will enter into an agreement with the VA to perform a certain number of hours of work in exchange for compensation. Eligible individuals may work for up to 25 hours times the number of weeks contained in an enrollment period. They receive the greater of the state's minimum wage rate or the national minimum wage rate under section 6(a) of the Fair Labor Standards Act of 1938 (Title 29 U.S.C. § 206(a)). Eligible work-study activities are

- outreach services to ensure that all veterans are provided timely and appropriate assistance to aid and encourage them in applying for and obtaining VA benefits,
- preparation and processing of necessary papers and other documents at educational institutions or regional offices or facilities of the VA,

- hospital and domiciliary care and medical treatment at VA facilities,
- activities related to the administration of MGIB-SR at DOD, Coast Guard, or National Guard facilities (for Reservists only), and
- any other appropriate activity of the VA.

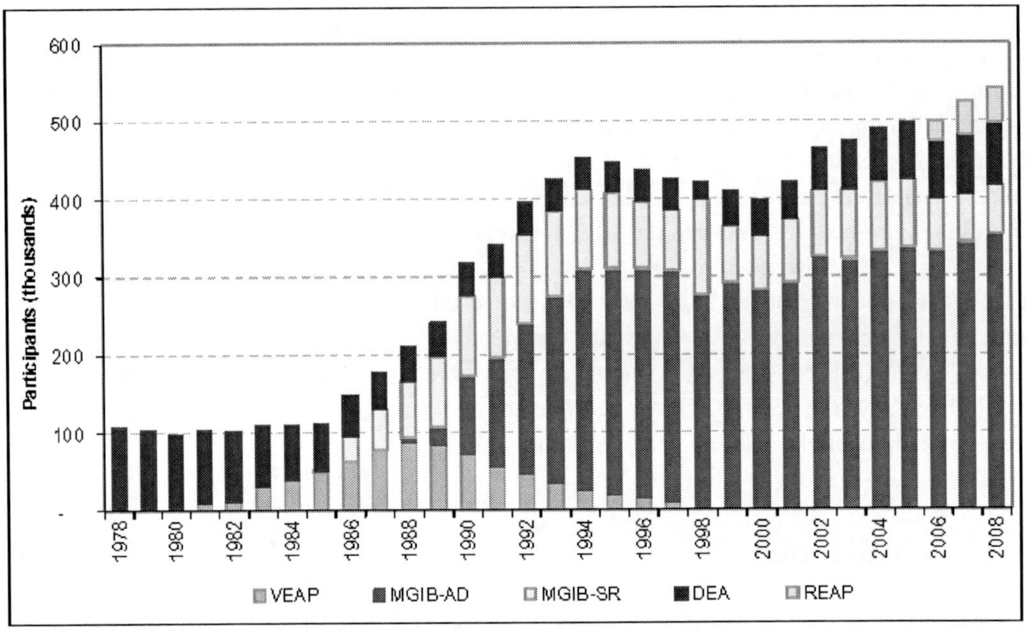

Source: Department of Veterans Affairs' Annual Reports 1978-1997 and data provided to CRS by the Department of Veterans Affairs, 1998-2008.

Notes: Beneficiaries may receive benefits in more than one year. The figure excludes concurrent participation in the Post-Korea and Vietnam Era GI Bill and the Veterans and Dependents Education Loan Program.

Figure 1. Total Veterans, Active-Duty Service Members, Reservists and Dependents Receiving VEAP, MGIB-AD, MGIB-SR, REAP, and DEA Education Benefits each Year (1978-2008)

Table 5. Undergraduate Veterans' Educational Assistance Recipients and Average Amount of Aid by Type of Military Service 2007-08 Academic year

	Percentage of undergraduates	Percentage receiving veterans' educational assistance	Average veterans' Educational assistance ($)
Total undergraduates	100	2.3	5,573
Veterans	3.1	38.3	6,138
Active duty military	0.7	38.5	4,167
Reservists	0.4	56.6	5,009
No military service	95.8	0.6	5,241

Source: CRS analysis based on U.S. Department of Education, National Center for Education Statistics, 2007– 2008 National Postsecondary Student Aid Study (NPSAS:08).

Notes: Military participation and the receipt of VA and DOD educational benefits during the 2007-2008 academic year are based on institutional records and self-reported information on federal financial aid applications and student interviews.

Table 6. Obligations and Participation of Selected Programs Administered by the VA: FY2008

Program	2008 Obligation ($ thousand)	Participation	2008 Appropriation per participant ($)
VEAP	746	560	1,333
MGIB-AD	2,112,635	354,284	5,984
MGIB-SR	149,344	62,403	2,393
REAP	148,580	44,025	3,375
DEA	434,715	80,191	5,421
VR&E Subsistence Allowance	238,131	55,059	4,325
VR&E Books, Tuition, Supplies, Fees, etc.	377,796	16,231	5,299

Source: Department of Veterans Affairs, *FY2010 Budget Submission*, pp. 2b-3 and 2d-4, http://www.va.gov/ budget/summary/20 1 0/Volume_3-Benefits_and_Burial_and_Dept_Admin .pdf.

Special provisions of the work-study program allow individuals to receive a lump sum advance payment after signing a contract to complete a certain number of work-study hours. The advance may be 40% of the expected allowance or 50 hours of earnings at the minimum wage rate, whichever is lower.

PARTICIPATION AND COST

Participation in VEAP, MGIBs, REAP, and DEA is exhibited in **Figure 1**. Participation in VEAP peaked in 1988 at 88,964 and is slowly declining as the eligible individuals become older or transfer to other programs. The number of participants in the MGIBs has been moderately stable since 1994 for MGIB-AD, nine years after implementation, and since 1989 for MGIB-SR, four years after implementation. Since individuals eligible to receive benefits under the MGIB-SR cannot receive benefits after separating from the Selected Reserves, it may be more important to initiate use of the benefits as soon as possible after initial eligibility. Also, the Reserve population may be more mature than the population first entering active duty such that their long-term plans are more likely to have been determined. MGIB-AD participation has averaged 310,000 since 1994. MGIB-SR participation has averaged 88,000 since 1989. Participation in REAP has increased in each of its three years, 2006 through 2008. Participation cycles in DEA mirror major conflicts with greater participation around the Vietnam Conflict, 1978-1982, and around the conflict in Iraq, 2004-2008.

Although the educational assistance programs administered by the VA provide a significant benefit to veterans and service members, the programs have very little impact on the total undergraduate population (**Table 5**). The programs served fewer than half of all veterans and service members in undergraduate postsecondary education in the 2007-2008 academic year. Fewer than 3% of undergraduates and about one-third of undergraduate veterans and active duty military personnel receive any veterans' educational assistance. The small percentage, less than 1%, of undergraduates with no military service who receive veterans' benefits may be in the DEA program, the MGIB-AD Army pilot program allowing the transfer of benefits to dependents, or a DOD program.

Table 6 compares participation and cost of selected programs administered by the VA. The program with the largest participation and obligations in FY2008 was the MGIB-AD, with almost 350,000 participants and total obligations of over $2.1 billion. The program with the smallest participation was VEAP, with 560 participants and total obligations of less than $1 million. The MGIB-AD program was more expensive at $5,984 per participant. In the FY2010 Budget, the VA estimates that participation in the Post-9/11 GI Bill will reach almost half of a million, at an average cost of $16,164 per participant, while the MGIB-AD participation will decrease to less than 50,000 as most participants transfer to the new program.

APPENDIX A. EDUCATIONAL ASSISTANCE UNDER THE ORIGINAL GI BILL OF RIGHTS[109]

The original GI Bill, the Servicemen's Readjustment Act of 1944 (P.L. 78-346), was intended to help veterans returning from World War II (WWII). The original GI Bill provided unprecedented benefits: funds to the VA to build and administer additional hospital facilities; extended vocational rehabilitation and employment services; educational assistance to non-disabled veterans; loans for the purchase or construction of homes, farms, and business property at advantageous terms to veterans; employment services to returning veterans; and unemployment benefits to veterans. The purpose of the educational assistance program was to avoid high levels of unemployment as had occurred following World War I, to help service members readjust to civilian life, and to afford returning veterans an opportunity to receive the education and training missed while providing compulsory service in the military.[110] From December 1, 1941, through December 31, 1946, 16.1 million personnel served in the U.S. armed forces in WWII.[111] The U.S. population in 1946 is estimated at 141,388,566.[112]

Eligible Individuals

Educational assistance benefits were available to all veterans who served on active duty in the military or naval service after September 16, 1940, and before the termination of WWII hostilities (December 31, 1946). Eligible veterans must have been discharged other than dishonorably and have served a minimum of 90 days or have been discharged or released for a service-incurred injury or disability. The 90-day service period excluded time spent completing the Army specialized training program or Navy college training program and excluded time spent as a cadet or midshipman at one of the service academies.

Benefit Availability and Duration of Use

Eligible veterans were required to begin an education program within two years of discharge or release or within two years of the end of WWII, whichever was later. The start date was later extended by P.L. 79-268, enacted in 1945, to four years after discharge or release or December 31, 1950, whichever was later. Veterans were entitled to at least one year of education (or the equivalent for continuous part-time study) or the length of the chosen education program if that program was shorter than 12 months. Upon satisfactory completion of the first year (or the period of a shorter education program), veterans whose education had been interrupted upon entering military service were entitled to educational benefits for at least as long as they served after September 16, 1940, and before the end of WWII, but not more than four years. The restriction, which provided no more than one year of educational benefits to certain veterans, was later removed to provide the same benefits to all veterans.[113] By law, no educational benefits under the original GI Bill could be paid seven years after the end of WWII, or July 25, 1956.[114]

Eligible Programs of Education, Institutions, and Establishments

Initially, the eligible educational institutions were almost any institutions providing education: public or private elementary, secondary, and other schools furnishing education for adults; business schools; scientific and technical institutions; colleges and universities; vocational schools; junior colleges; teachers' colleges; professional schools; and other educational institutions. The eligible training establishments were businesses or other establishments offering apprentice or on-the-job training. Because the quality of some training programs was poor, laws were enacted establishing approval criteria for training institutions and for-profit schools.[115] Stricter criteria were prescribed for on-the-job and on-the-farm training programs and vocational schools.[116] Also, avocational and recreational training programs, such as nonvocational flight training, were eventually prohibited.[117]

Benefit Payments

Under the GI Bill, the VA paid up to $500 a year directly to an educational institution for tuition, books, fees, and other training costs for each enrolled veteran. Institutions providing apprentice or on-the-job training did not receive this payment. Veterans were required to maintain satisfactory conduct or progress in their chosen program of education. To increase flexibility, the program was revised by P.L. 79-268, enacted in 1945, to allow veterans to receive higher annual tuition and fees payments (accelerated payments) for a corresponding reduction in the period of entitlement.

The VA also paid up to $50 monthly as a subsistence allowance to single veterans, and $75 monthly to veterans with one or more dependents. The monthly payment was eventually increased to $75 monthly for single veterans, $105 monthly for veterans with one dependent, and $120 monthly for veterans with more than one dependent by P.L. 80-411, enacted in 1948. Veterans who attended part-time or received compensation for apprentice or on-the-job training received a lower subsistence allowance. In 1945, P.L. 79-268 specifically authorized tuition and fees payments for correspondence courses but disallowed the subsistence allowance. Later, P.L. 79-679, enacted in 1946, limited total earnings for veterans receiving compensation for apprentice or on-the-job training. Veterans were limited to a total monthly employment compensation plus VA subsistence allowance of no more than $175 for single veterans and $200 for veterans with dependents. This was increased to $210 for single veterans, $270 for veterans with one dependent, and $290 for veterans with more than one dependent by P.L. 80-512, enacted in 1948.

Lessons Learned

Some important lessons were learned in the implementation of the original GI Bill, and as the result of several studies.[118] Paying tuition and fees directly to educational institutions led to overpayments and excessive payments to for-profit vocational training programs in particular.[119] Some institutions were created solely to profit from the program.[120] It was necessary to define and establish standards for the eligible training establishments and educational institutions to ensure adequate quality of the educational programs and to define and remunerate responsibility for evaluating them.[121] There was considerable objection to the use of the GI Bill for avocational and recreational purposes since one of the stated purposes of the program was workforce preparation.[122] The third mechanism for ensuring proper use of the GI Bill educational assistance was the importance placed on veterans' identifying and adhering to an educational objective. Finally, it was necessary to increase the benefits as the cost of living and education increased.

Participation and Costs

In the end, the nation spent $14.5 billion ($114.7 billion in 2008 inflation adjusted dollars) to provide education and training to 7.8 million WWII veterans (**Table A-1**).[123] The total expenditure per participant was $1,859 ($14,700 in 2008 inflation adjusted dollars).

Table A- 1. Original GI Bill Participation

	Number
Veteran Population	15,440,000
Total trained	7,800,000
College and other school trainees	5,710,000
College trainees	2,230,000
Other school trainees	3,480,000
On-the-job trainees	1,400,000
On-the-farm trainees	690,000

Source: Veterans Administration, *Veterans Benefits under Current Educational Programs, Fiscal Year 1984*, Washington, 1984, p. 28.

APPENDIX B. KOREAN CONFLICT GI BILL[124]

The Veterans' Readjustment Assistance Act of 1952 (P.L. 82-550, also known as the Korean Conflict GI Bill) was authorized to help veterans returning from the Korean Conflict adjust to civilian life. The program was codified in Title 38 U.S.C., Chapter 33, before its subsequent repeal. The expected number of Korean Conflict veterans, less than six million (or 4%) of a national population of 157,552,740 in 1952,[125] was lower than the number of WWII veterans, reducing the risk of high national unemployment in comparison to the post-WWI and post-WWII eras. The Korean Conflict GI Bill was intended to provide veterans the education forestalled by compulsory service and provide equitable benefits, as had been afforded the WWII veterans. The bill was also written in an effort to avoid many problems encountered in the implementation of the original GI Bill. [126]

Eligible Individuals

Veteran eligibility was essentially the same for the Korean GI Bill as the original GI Bill except that only those armed forces who served on active duty during the Korean Conflict (on or after June 27, 1950, and before the termination of hostilities on January 31, 1955[127]) were eligible. Veterans still had to be discharged other than dishonorably and serve a minimum of 90 days, or discharged or released for a service-incurred injury or disability. The 90-day service period excluded time assigned to an education or training program similar to those offered to civilians and excluded time spent as a cadet or midshipman at one of the service academies.

Benefit Availability and Duration of Use

While WWII veterans were afforded up to four years of education benefits, Korean Conflict veterans were limited to 36 months, which is substantially equivalent for students attending traditional postsecondary schools with summers off. Eligible veterans were required to begin an education program within two years (later extended to three years by P.L. 83-6 10, enacted in 1954) of discharge or release or before August 21, 1954, whichever was later. Veterans were entitled to educational benefits for a period equal to 1½ times the duration of their active duty service between June 27, 1950, and the termination of hostilities, but no more than 36 months. Veterans enrolled entirely in correspondence courses were entitled to educational benefits for a period equal to six times the duration of their active duty service. Veterans could combine benefits with the VR&E program or the original GI Bill to receive up to 48 months of educational benefits. By law, no educational benefits under the Korean Conflict GI Bill could be paid seven years after discharge or release or upon the termination of hostilities, whichever was earlier.[128]

This was later extended to eight years after discharge or release or January 31, 1965, by P.L. 84-7, enacted in 1955.

Table B- 1. Korean Conflict GI Bill Participation

	Number
Veteran Population	5,509,000
Total trained	2,391,000
College and other school trainees	2,073,000
College trainees	1,213,000
Other school trainees	860,000
On-the-job trainees	223,000
On-the-farm trainees	95,000

Source: Veterans Administration, *Veterans Benefits under Current Educational Programs, Fiscal Year 1984*, Washington, 1984, p. 28.

Eligible Programs of Education, Institutions, and Establishments

The list of eligible educational institutions and training establishments did not change from the original GI Bill except that institutions listed on the Attorney General's List of Subversive Organizations[129] were not eligible. States were requested to create state approving agencies to approve educational courses and provide lists of eligible institutions. The VA provided some cost reimbursement of salaries and travel for these state agencies.

To ensure the benefits were used for workforce preparation and to avoid some of the misuse experienced under the original GI Bill, several provisions were added or changed from the original GI Bill. Veterans were required to declare an educational objective or certificate/degree. They were allowed to change their educational objective only once, only if not making satisfactory progress by no fault of misconduct, neglect, or lack of application, and if the new program fit their aptitude or previous education or the new program was a normal progression from the existing program. The legislation specifically prohibited veterans from receiving benefits for avocational and recreational courses in bartending, dance, photography, music, sports, and personal development.[130]

The criteria and standards for approving training establishments and educational institutions were bolstered in comparison to the original GI Bill. Veterans could not enroll in non-accredited courses below the college level at institutions that received more than 85% of their funding from the VA through either the VR&E or the original GI Bill. Substantially new courses at private institutions (later applied to only private for-profit institutions by P.L. 84-847, enacted in 1956) that had been offered for fewer than two years were not eligible to veterans. Amendments to the original GI Bill establishing stringent standards for apprentice, on-the-job, and on-the-farm training were expanded under the Korean Conflict GI Bill to include courses already approved by nationally recognized accrediting agencies and certain courses without accreditation.

Benefit Payments

The Korean Conflict GI Bill made payments only to veterans, as opposed to the payments made to veterans and educational institutions under the original GI Bill. The U.S. House of Representatives' Select Committee to Investigate Educational, Training, and Loan Guaranty Programs under the GI Bill (1950-1952) indicated that direct payments to educational institutions led to abuse.[131] A 1956 House Report determined that because the original GI Bill was generous, some veterans used the benefits for income rather than to achieve an employment goal.[132] It was also believed that if veterans were responsible for paying a portion of the cost of their own education that this, in combination with the payment of benefits directly to veterans, would encourage more careful spending.[133]

Since maximum benefits were offered to veterans in full-time study, the legislation provided a uniform definition of full-time for below college-level trade, technical, and institutional courses offered on the clock-hour basis and for undergraduate courses offered at colleges and universities. The benefit provided an allowance for subsistence, tuition, fees, supplies, books, and equipment of up to $110 monthly to single veterans, $135 monthly to veterans with one dependent, and $160 monthly to veterans with more than one dependent. Veterans who attended institutional training less then full-time, attended on-the-farm training at least half-time, or attended cooperative training full-time received a lower allowance. As a result of the determination that some veterans were overpaid from the original GI Bill,[134] veterans who attended apprentice or on-the-job training received an allowance, which could not exceed $310 monthly in combination with the veterans' employment compensation. Veterans completing all coursework through correspondence courses or on a less-than-half-time basis were only reimbursed for the cost of completed courses. Veterans in flight training received 75% of the cost of flight training unless the program of education combined flight training with other coursework.[135]

An allowance was not paid if veterans were absent from unaccredited courses or apprentice or on- the-job training for more than 30 days. Veterans could not suspend their education for longer than 12 months without a waiver from the VA. Veterans and their institutions were required to certify attendance, lessons completed, and/or satisfactory progress. The law disallowed veterans from receiving duplicate benefits from the Korean Conflict GI Bill and any other educational benefit from the U.S. Treasury.

Participation and Cost

In the end, the nation spent $4.5 billion ($30.8 billion in 2008 inflation adjusted dollars) to provide education and training to almost 2.4 million Korean Conflict veterans (**Table B-1**). The total expenditure per participant was $1,882 ($12,867 in 2008 inflation adjusted dollars).

Appendix C. Post-Korea and Vietnam Era GI Bill[136]

Once fighting and ground troop deployment escalated in Vietnam, the Veterans Readjustment Benefits Act of 1966 (P.L. 89-358), better known as the Post-Korea and

Vietnam Era[137] GI Bill, was passed. The program is codified in Title 38 U.S.C., Chapter 34. Congress passed the bill unanimously despite reservations by President Lyndon B. Johnson that the cost was too high.[138] The benefits were designed to help recruit new service members, extend benefits to all who fulfilled their compulsory service, and afford returning veterans an opportunity to receive the education and training missed while providing compulsory service in the military. Although the benefits were initially intended to provide "considerably less liberal treatment" to non-war veterans,[139] over time Congress expanded the benefits and liberalized eligibility. Incidentally, these veterans were eligible for other federal education benefits available to the general public and passed through the recently enacted Higher Education Act of 1965.

Eligible Individuals

The new GI Bill increased the minimum active duty eligibility from 90 days, as in the original and Korean Conflict GI Bills, to 180 days and made service members eligible for benefits while on active duty. Educational assistance benefits were available to all veterans who served on active-duty after January 31, 1955, who were discharged other than dishonorably and served a minimum of 180 days, or were discharged or released for a service-connected disability. The 180- day service period excluded time assigned to an education or training program similar to those offered to civilians, time spent as a cadet or midshipman at one of the service academies, time spent in college for a delayed enlistment in the Army National Guard or Air National Guard, and service in the National Guard and Reserves. The program was later amended by P.L. 93-508, enacted in 1974, so that members of the National Guard and Reserves after the initial active duty training period were eligible if the active duty period was at least one year.

Service members remaining on active duty were eligible to use the benefits after serving two continuous years on active duty. This provision responded to concerns by the DOD that benefits available to veterans only would be counter to retention efforts.[140]

Benefit Availability and Duration of Use

Although the bill was not passed until 1966, the benefits retroactively covered active duty servicemen since 1955 such that there would be no period of ineligibility of educational assistance benefits since September 16, 1940. Unlike the Korean Conflict GI Bill, there was no timeframe in which eligible persons had to begin an educational program. By law, no educational benefits under the Post-Korean Conflict GI Bill could be paid eight years (later extended to ten years by P.L. 93-337, enacted in 1974) after discharge or release or eight years after the Bill's enactment, whichever was later.[141]

Although Korean Conflict veterans were entitled to educational benefits for a period equal to 1½ times the duration of their active duty, this was initially reduced in the Post-Korean Conflict GI Bill to one month for each month of active duty service, but still no more than 36 months. P.L. 90-631, enacted in 1968, increased the period of entitlement to 1½ months of benefits for every month of service, with those serving 18 months or more being entitled to the full 36 months of benefits (the same formula that had applied to the Korean Conflict GI Bill). Later, the entitlement period was increased to 45 months for those pursuing a standard undergraduate college degree by P.L. 93-508, enacted in 1974, and finally to 45 months for all eligible persons by P.L. 94-502, enacted in 1976. Although Korean Conflict GI Bill veterans could combine benefits with other educational benefit programs administered by the VA to receive up to 48 months of educational benefits, this was originally reduced to 36 months under the Post-Korean Conflict GI Bill, but increased back to 48 months by P.L. 90-631, enacted in 1968. P.L. 94-502, enacted in 1976, terminated eligibility for those entering military service after December 31, 1976, and provided that no educational benefits could be paid after December 31, 1989.

Eligible Programs of Education, Institutions, and Establishments

Many of the provisions initiated in the Korean Conflict GI Bill to ensure the benefits were used to promote quality work force preparation were maintained. Benefit recipients were required to declare an educational, professional, or vocational objective; however, there was greater latitude to change the objective.[142] Avocational and recreational courses were still disallowed. [143] No allowance was paid if veterans were absent from courses, which did not lead to a standard college degree, for more than 30 days. Substantially new courses at private for-profit institutions that had been offered for fewer than two years were not eligible.

New provisions to ensure proper use of funds were added. Flight training courses had to be offered by IHLs and lead to a standard college degree (later revised to the standard college degree the recipient was seeking by P.L. 90-77, enacted in 1967). No on-the-job or on-the-farm course (later expanded to any course by P.L. 90-77, enacted in 1967) could be offered through open circuit television or radio, and no program of education leading to a standard college degree could offer the majority of courses through open circuit television or radio. Benefit recipients could not enroll in unaccredited courses below the college level at private institutions at which more than 85% of the students received payments from the institution or the VA. Disclosure and refund requirements for correspondence schools were prescribed to fight low completion rates by P.L. 92-540, enacted in 1972. P.L. 97-306, enacted in 1982, added provisions that payments could be suspended for courses where there was a substantial pattern of ineligible trainees receiving assistance because course approval requirements had not been met or the institution offering the course had violated recordkeeping requirements. Programs of education outside the United States were allowed only if offered at approved IHLs.

The list of eligible educational institutions and training establishments was initially narrowed from the Korean Conflict GI Bill to exclude public or private elementary schools, other schools furnishing education for adults, and businesses or other establishments offering apprenticeships or on-the-job training. These institutions and establishments were later added back to the list. The State Approving Agencies were maintained from the Korean Conflict GI Bill. Educational institutions were still required to report enrollment, interruption, and termination of education to the VA, but would start receiving an annual reporting fee for each eligible person[144] receiving educational benefits from the VA.

Eligibility and requirements were later added for small business, farm cooperative, on-the-job training (excluding apprenticeship), and flight training establishments to receive approval as eligible educational institutions from the State Approving Agency. Courses required by the Small Business Administration as a condition for obtaining financial assistance became eligible under P.L. 91-584, enacted in 1970. Farm cooperative training requiring 12 weekly hours of institutional agricultural courses and relevant agricultural employment became eligible under P.L. 90-77, enacted in 1967. P.L. 90-77 also provided strict requirements for on-the-job training programs: requiring progression and appointment to the next highest level based on the skills learned as opposed to length of service; providing compensation that matched non-veterans; providing initial compensation of not less than 50% of the final, full wage; requiring a reasonable guarantee that the job would be available upon completion of the training period; qualifying the trainee for the job; requiring at least six months of training but no more than two years; and requiring adequate resources for the training. Flight training eligibility was allowed by P.L. 90-77, enacted in 1967, for the attainment of a vocational objective in aviation for those with a valid private pilot's license or sufficient flight training hours for a private pilot's license (the allowance of sufficient hours without a license was later deleted by P.L. 91-219, enacted in 1970) if the flight school was approved by the State Approving Agency and Federal Aviation Administration. However, flight training for new enrollees was terminated by P.L. 97-35, enacted in 1981.

Benefit Payments

Like the Korean Conflict GI Bill, an allowance for subsistence, tuition and fees, supplies, books, and equipment was paid directly to recipients. Veterans and service members received up to $150 monthly (eventually increased to $510 for individuals with two dependents) according to a schedule based on full-time,[145] three-quarter-time, or half-time or cooperative program enrollment and the number of dependents. Active duty service members and students pursuing education on a less-than-half-time basis were only reimbursed for the cost of completed courses, but no more than $100 monthly (eventually increased to $376 by P.L. 98-543, enacted in 1984). Students completing all coursework through correspondence courses were only reimbursed for the cost (eventually reduced to 55% of cost by P.L. 97-3 5, enacted in 1981) of completed courses, and their entitlement period was reduced by one quarter of the time in the program (eventually changed to one month of entitlement for each $376 reimbursed by P.L. 98-543, enacted in 1984). Veterans in full-time on-the-farm, apprentice, or on-the-job training received a reduced allowance. [146] In general, veterans and service members and their institutions were required to certify actual attendance, lessons completed, and/or satisfactory progress before payments were made.

Allowance and entitlement period provisions were added for students pursuing a standard college degree through independent study and for students pursuing education while incarcerated or in a half-way house by P.L. 96-466, enacted in 1980. The law disallowed veterans from receiving duplicate educational benefits from the U.S. Treasury.

For the first time, after the enactment of P.L. 91-219 in 1970, veterans and service members were allowed to receive an advance payment for the first month of enrollment only. P.L. 95-202, enacted in 1977, authorized the state or local government to establish a program with the VA that would allow veterans to use accelerated payments to help repay certain VA loans. The veteran had to be enrolled full-time and complete the program satisfactorily with a degree, diploma, or certificate. The tuition and fees had to exceed $700 for a term, and no more than 35% of program students could have received VA benefits. If these requirements were met, the state or local government paid the VA a matching amount of the accelerated payment.

Predischarge Education Program

The Predischarge Education Program (PREP) allowed service members who completed 180 days of active duty and were still on active duty to receive an allowance for non-correspondence courses leading to a high school diploma or any deficiency, remedial, or refresher course in preparation for enrollment in an approved educational institution or training establishment. The monthly allowance was the lesser of actual tuition, fees, books, and supplies or $175 (eventually increased to $270 by P.L. 93-602, enacted in 1975). Allowances received while on active duty did not reduce the regular entitlement period upon discharge or release.[147]

Training for the Educationally Disadvantaged

The Post-Korean Conflict GI Bill was later amended to provide special assistance and training for the educationally disadvantaged. First, P.L. 90-77, enacted in 1967, allowed veterans and service members without a high school diploma or its equivalent or who needed additional secondary school courses to receive the regular allowance for these courses without the payments reducing their regular entitlement period. Second, P.L. 91-219, enacted in 1970, provided tutorial assistance of $50 monthly for nine months (eventually increased to $84 monthly for a maximum of 12 months, or $1,008, by P.L. 98-543, enacted in 1984) to veterans and service members enrolled in postsecondary education at least half-time. The tutorial assistance had to be for a deficiency in a course required for the educational objective, and the educational institution had to certify the need for assistance, the qualifications of the tutor, and the customary nature of the charges. Receipt of tutorial assistance did not reduce their regular entitlement period under the Post-Korean Conflict GI Bill.

Work-Study

P.L. 92-540, enacted in 1972, created a veteran work-study allowance for full-time students (later liberalized to at least three-quarter-time students by P.L. 101-237, enacted in 1989). The allowance of $250 or a prorated sum (eventually increased to minimum wage or $625, whichever is higher, by P.L. 95-202, enacted in 1977) was paid based on the agreement of a veteran to perform 100 hours of work in a term (eventually increased to a number of hours equal to 25 times the number of weeks in the term by P.L. 101-237, enacted in 1989). Eligible work was VA outreach services, preparation and processing of paperwork at the educational institution or VA, medical care, or other activities approved by the VA. Preference was given to veterans with greater than 30% disability.

APPENDIX D. VETERANS AND DEPENDENTS EDUCATION LOAN PROGRAM[148]

The Veterans and Dependents Education Loan Program was established by the Vietnam Era Veterans' Readjustment Assistance Act of 1974 (P.L. 93-508) in Chapter 36 of Title 38 U.S.C. to provide additional support to veterans attending high-cost institutions. Veterans who served on active duty after January 31, 1955, and before January 1, 1977 (later modified to active duty after January 31, 1955, by P.L. 94-502, enacted in 1976), and their spouses, widows, and children were eligible to borrow. Eligible individuals also had to be enrolled at least half-time in a program of education leading to a standard college degree or a six-month non-college degree. Loans were not eligible for correspondence courses or apprentice and on-the-job training. Veterans who were full- time students were allowed loans for another two years of their remaining dollars of entitlement once the VEAP entitlement period ended. Repayment began nine months after enrollment dropped below half-time and was completed within ten years.

The loans were up to $600 (eventually increased to $2,500 by P.L. 95-202, enacted in 1977) annually for education expenses. They were expected to cover the difference between the cost of attendance and the individual's reasonable financial resources.

There were several problems with the program's administration. The majority of loans were initially made to individuals at no- or low-cost institutions until P.L. 95-476 specified high-cost institutions. The loans were made without regard to other financial assistance such as Department of Education student financial assistance programs. The financial needs of 99% of recipients could have been covered through Department of Education student financial assistance programs. The default rate increased from 44% as of December 31, 1997, to 65% as of September 30, 1980. It also cost the VA 70 times more to administer the program than the Department of Education. P.L. 97-35 repealed the VA education loan program as of September 30, 1981, with some exceptions.[149,150]

End Notes

[1] References to DOD include the Department of Homeland Security with respect to the Coast Guard when it is not operating as a service in the Navy.

[2] Edward Humes, "The Greatest Generation: The Accidental Remaking of America," in *Over Here: How the G.I. Bill Transformed the American Dream*, 1st ed. (Orlando, FL: Harcourt, Inc., 2006), pp. 4-20.

[3] Suzanne Metler, *Soldiers to Citizens: The G.I. Bill and the Making of the Greatest Generation* (New York: Oxford University Press, 2005), p. 26.

[4] Facts for Features, U.S. Census Bureau, April 29, 2004, http://www.census.gov/Press-Release/www/2004/cb04-ffse07.pdf.

[5] The Armed Forces are the Army, Navy, Air Force, Marine Corps, and Coast Guard of the United States.

[6] U.S. Census Bureau, Table 1. Years of School Completed by Persons 14 Years Old and Over, by Age, Color, and Sex, for the United States: Civilian Population, April 1947, and Total Population, April 1940.

[7] The American Legion was chartered by Congress in 1919 as a patriotic wartime veterans organization devoted to mutual helpfulness. It is a not-for-profit community-service organization.

[8] Correspondence training differs from distance learning or online education in that individuals in correspondence training usually receive lessons in the mail and have a certain amount of time to complete and return them for a grade.

[9] U.S. Congress, Senate Committee on Veterans' Affairs, *Veterans Education and Employment Assistance Act of 1976*, Hearings before the Subcommittee on Readjustment, Education, and Employment of the Committee on Veterans Affairs on S. 969 and Related Bills, 94th Cong., 1st sess., October 1, 1975, S. Rept 761-4.

[10] Certain individuals in the Armed Forces who receive educational assistance or other benefits are required to serve an obligated period of active duty or repay a portion of the benefit.

[11] The National Guard includes the Army National Guard and Air National Guard.

[12] In certain circumstances, individuals on active duty could make a lump-sum contribution in lieu of or in addition to the monthly payments. The lump-sum payment is counted as if the individual made $100 monthly contributions.

[13] Individuals on active duty could re-enroll at any time before July 1, 1985.

[14] Veterans who are incapable of beginning education as a result of a physical or mental disability can be granted an extension for the period of incapacity.

[15] A cooperative program is a full-time program of education, which consists of institutional courses and alternate phases of training in a business or industrial establishment with the training in a business or industrial establishment being strictly supplemental.

[16] All programs of education must be approved by the VA and other relevant approving agencies.

[17] To calculate an individual's monthly allowance, the individual's contributions are multiplied by three, the DOD contributions are added to the result, and the sum is divided by the lesser of the number of months of contributions or 36.

[18] Veterans benefits cannot duplicate those paid under any other federal, state, or local program.

[19] Established charges are the lesser of the charge for the course(s) determined on the basis of the lowest extended time payment plan offered by the institution and approved by the appropriate State Approving Agency or the tuition and fees or charges that similarly circumstanced nonveterans enrolled in the same course(s) are required to pay. Individuals may only receive payment for the minimum number of solo flying hours required by the Federal Aviation Administration for the desired flight rating or certification. For exclusive flight training, an individual's entitlement period is reduced one month for each amount paid that is equal to the monthly benefit otherwise payable to such individual.

[20] For licensing, certification, admissions, or course credit testing, an individual's entitlement period is reduced one month for each amount paid that is equal to the monthly benefit otherwise payable to such individual.

[21] For apprentice or on-the-job training, an individual's entitlement period is respectively reduced 0.75, 0.55, or 0.35 months for each month of educational assistance, depending on the payment. Individuals working/training fewer than 120 hours monthly have their payment and entitlement period usage proportionately reduced.

[22] Honorable Bob Edgar indicated in his prepared statement that "up to an estimated one-third of active duty male first term enlistees from fiscal year 1976 to fiscal year 1978 failed to complete three years of initial service." U.S. Congress, House Committee on Armed Services, Subcommittee on Military Personnel and Compensation, *New Educational Assistance Program for the Military to Assist Recruiting*, 97th Cong., 1st and 2nd sess., June 24, September 10, 16, 17, 24, 30, October 1, 7, 21, 28, November 17, 1981, and March 11, 1982, HRG-1981-ASH-0030 (Washington: GPO, 1982).

[23] U.S. Congress, House Committee on Armed Services, Subcommittee on Military Personnel and Compensation, *New Educational Assistance Program for the Military to Assist Recruiting*, 97th Cong., 1st and 2nd sess., June 24, September 10, 16, 17, 24, 30, October 1, 7, 21, 28, November 17, 1981, and March 11, 1982, HRG-1981-ASH-0030 (Washington: GPO, 1982).

[24] The New GI Bill Continuation Act (P.L. 100-48) permanently authorized the All-Volunteer Force Educational Assistance Program and the Selected Reserve Component. It also changed the name of the program to the Montgomery GI Bill.

[25] Secretary of Defense Melvin Laird introduced the Total Force Concept of the Armed Forces in 1970 to reduce military expenditures by calling on the Reserves and National Guard to serve an increased active duty role.

[26] U.S. Congress, House Committee on Armed Services, Subcommittee on Military Personnel and Compensation, *New Educational Assistance Program for the Military to Assist Recruiting*, 97th Cong., 1st and 2nd sess., June 24, September 10, 16, 17, 24, 30, October 1, 7, 21, 28, November 17, 1981, and March 11, 1982, H.A.S.C. 97-45 (Washington: GPO, 1982).

[27] Individuals eligible for the Post-Korean Conflict GI Bill who have been on continuous active duty since October 19, 1984, and served at least three years of continuous active duty after June 30, 1985, or were discharged or released from active duty after June 30, 1985, for a service-connected disability or hardship, or were discharged for the government's convenience after serving a minimum of 30 months active duty after June 30, 1985, are also eligible to MGIB-AD educational benefits. Category 2 individuals also include Reservists eligible for the Post-Korean Conflict GI Bill who serve two continuous years of honorable active duty service in the military after June 30, 1985, and who serve a minimum of four continuous years of service in the Reserves immediately following the active duty service. Category 2 includes individuals eligible for the Post-

Korean Conflict GI Bill who were not on active duty on October 19, 1984, but re-enlisted and served three continuous years on active duty or were discharged or released for reasons similar to those of other individuals eligible for the Post-Korean Conflict GI Bill.

[28] Selected Reservists may make a one-time lump-sum contribution or 12-monthly contributions totaling $1,200 after completing two years of active duty service. In the event of an individual's service-connected death while on active duty, the designated beneficiary, surviving spouse, children, or parents will be reimbursed any contribution by the service member that had not already been used.

[29] Service members were allowed to withdraw their election to not enroll in the program during an open period between December 1, 1988, and June 30, 1989; before being involuntarily separated; and before separating from the active service with an honorable discharge and receiving certain voluntary separation incentives.

[30] Veterans who were ineligible for the program on discharge or release but whose discharge status was later amended to make them eligible for the program are allowed benefits for up to 10 years after the discharge status was amended. The 10-year period excludes periods detained by a foreign government or power and any recovery period in a hospital. Veterans who were incapable of beginning education as a result of a physical or mental disability could be granted an extension for the period of incapacity. The 10-year period is reduced for individuals eligible for the Post-Korean Conflict GI Bill by the length of time not on active duty service between January 1, 1977, and October 18, 1984. Also, the 10-year period begins after discharge or release from active duty or on January 1, 1990, whichever is later, for Post- Korean Conflict GI Bill participants who were on active duty after October 18, 1984. For Post-Korean Conflict GI Bill participants who were not on active duty on October 19, 1984, the 10-year period begins on December 27, 2001.

[31] Reservists who are discharged or released with a service-connected disability or pre-existing medical condition during the four-year Reserve period are eligible for 36 months of educational assistance.

[32] Prior to FY20 10, the maximum monthly benefit amounts could be adjusted at any time by Congress or be adjusted annually according to the consumer price index for all urban consumers (CPI-U).

[33] Snyder, T.D., Dillow, S.A., and Hoffman, C.M., *Digest of Education Statistics 2008* (NCES 2009-020), National Center for Education Statistics, Institute of Education Sciences, U.S. Department of Education, Washington, DC, 2009, pp. 474-476.

[34] The benefit payment has been increased several times since the program's enactment. When the MGIB-AD program was enacted in 1985, the maximum monthly benefit was $300. The maximum monthly benefit was increased to $400 by the Veterans' Benefits Act of 1992 (P.L. 102-568), to $528 by the Transportation Equity Act for the 21st Century (P.L. 105-178) in 1998, and to $650 by the Veterans Benefits and Health Care Improvement Act of 2000 (P.L. 106- 419). The Veterans Education and Benefits Expansion Act of 2001 (P.L. 107-103) provided three increases: $800 for months beginning on or after January 1, 2002; $900 for months occurring during FY2003; and $985 for months occurring during FY2004. For FY2009, the monthly benefit amount was increased to $1,321 by the Supplemental Appropriations Act, 2008 (P.L. 110-252).

[35] For apprentice or on-the-job training, an individual's entitlement period is respectively reduced at 0.75, 0.55, or 0.35 months for each month of educational assistance received, depending on the payment. Individuals working/training fewer than 120 hours monthly have their payment and entitlement period usage proportionately reduced.

[36] The individual's entitlement period is reduced at 0.8 months for each month of cooperative educational assistance received.

[37] The individual's entitlement period is reduced one month for each educational assistance payment that equals the monthly assistance allowance to which the individual would have been entitled. Individuals may only receive payment for the minimum number of solo flying hours required by the Federal Aviation Administration for the desired flight rating or certification.

[38] For licensing, certification, admissions, or course credit testing, an individual's entitlement period is reduced one month for each amount paid that is equal to the monthly benefit otherwise payable to such individual.

[39] Upon completing the additional years of active duty service and Selected Reserves service, if applicable, the individual must remain on active duty; be discharged honorably; be placed on the retired or temporary disability retired list, or be transferred to the Reserves.

[40] The individual's entitlement period is reduced at a rate determined by dividing the amount of the Top-Up payment by the individual's full-time monthly rate.

[41] Children are defined as unmarried persons under the age of 18, unmarried persons who became permanently incapable of self-support before the age of 18, or unmarried persons between the ages of 18 and 23 who are in school. Children must be legitimate children, acknowledged illegitimate children, legally adopted, or stepchildren who are members of the eligible individual's household.

[42] Procedures and Guidance: Transfer of Montgomery G.I. Bill (MGIB) Benefits to Dependents: Expanded Army Pilot Program, November 1, 2007, at http://www.gibill.va.gov/documents/Army_Transferability_to_Dependents.pdf.

[43] Honorable Pete Geren and General George W. Casey, Jr., *A Statement on the Posture of the United States Army 2009*, United States Army, Transferability of GI Bill Benefits to Family Members, May 2009, http://www.army.mil/ aps/09/information_papers/transferability_bill_benefits.html.

[44] The Selected Reserves are generally required to participate in at least 48 scheduled drills or training periods during each year and serve on active duty for training for at least 14 days annually. See CRS Report RL3 0802, *Reserve Component Personnel Issues: Questions and Answers*, by Lawrence Kapp.

[45] The MGIB-SR program is codified under Title 10 U.S.C., Chapter 1606 (10 U.S.C. § 16131 et seq.).

[46] U.S. Congress, House Committee on Armed Services, Subcommittee on Military Personnel and Compensation, *New Educational Assistance Program for the Military To Assist Recruiting*, 97th Cong., 1st sess., June 24, 1981, HRG-198 1- ASH-0030, p. 70.

[47] Individuals receiving financial assistance under the Senior Reserve Officers' Training Corps are not eligible.

[48] Section 115(a) of Title 10 U.S.C. authorizes the number of military members in every branch and component. This number is known as *end strength*.

[49] Educational assistance would not end on separation if it was an involuntary separation or resulted from a disability that was not the result of the individual's own willful misconduct, the inactivation of the individual's unit during certain time periods, or other involuntary reasons. Individuals who were incapable of beginning education as a result of a physical or mental disability could be granted an extension for the period of incapacity.

[50] For apprentice or on-the-job training, an individual's entitlement period is respectively reduced 0.75, 0.55, or 0.35 months for each month of educational assistance, depending on the payment. Individuals working/training fewer than 120 hours monthly have their payment and entitlement period usage proportionately reduced.

[51] The entitlement period is reduced one month for every amount paid that is equal to the regular full-time monthly allowance. Individuals may only receive payment for the minimum number of solo flying hours required by the Federal Aviation Administration for the desired flight rating or certification.

[52] The entitlement period is reduced by the number of months equaling the proportion that the assistance is to the regular full-time monthly allowance.

[53] The transferred benefits could not be considered marital property in divorce proceedings.

[54] 10 U.S.C. § 16161 et seq.

[55] Individuals receiving financial assistance under the Senior Reserve Officers' Training Corps are not eligible.

[56] Individuals who were incapable of beginning education as a result of a physical or mental disability could be granted an extension for the period of incapacity.

[57] See CRS Report RL30802, *Reserve Component Personnel Issues: Questions and Answers*, by Lawrence Kapp.

[58] Based on rates effective October 1, 2009.

[59] The entitlement period is reduced by the number of months equaling the proportion that the assistance is to the regular full-time monthly allowance.

[60] The transferred benefits could not be considered marital property in divorce proceedings.

[61] Title IV of the Higher Education Act of 1965, as amended, authorizes several student aid programs: Pell Grant program, Federal Family Education Loan (FFEL) Program, William D. Ford Federal Direct Loan (DL) Program, American Competitiveness Grant program, National Science and Mathematics Access to Retain Talent (SMART) Grant program, Federal Supplemental Educational Opportunity Grant (FSEOG) program, Leveraging Educational Assistance Partnership (LEAP) program, Federal Work-Study (FWS) program, Federal Perkins Loan program, and Grants for Access and Persistence (GAP) program. See CRS Report RL34654, *The Higher Education Opportunity Act: Reauthorization of the Higher Education Act*, by David P. Smole et al.

[62] U.S. Congress, House Committee on Veterans' Affairs, Subcommittee on Economic Opportunity, *Pending Montgomery GI Bill Legislation*, 110th Cong., 2nd sess., January 17, 2008, HRG-2008-VAH-0003 (Washington: GPO, 2008), pp. 3, 6, 9, 10, 14 and U.S. Congress, Senate Committee on Veterans' Affairs, *Hearing on Pending Benefits Legislation*, 1 10th Cong., 2nd sess., May 7, 2008, S. Hrg. 110-675 (Washington: GPO, 2008), pp. 15, 21, 34, 49.

[63] U.S. Congress, House Committee on Veterans' Affairs, Subcommittee on Economic Opportunity, *Pending Montgomery GI Bill Legislation*, 1 10th Cong., 2nd sess., January 17, 2008, HRG-2008-VAH-0003 (Washington: GPO, 2008), pp. 3, 6, 9, 10, 14; and U.S. Congress, Senate Committee on Veterans' Affairs, *Hearing on Pending Benefits Legislation*, 1 10th Cong., 2nd sess., May 7, 2008, S. Hrg. 110-675 (Washington: GPO, 2008), pp. 15, 21, 34, 49.

[64] If the period of active duty service including entry level and skill training is at least 24 months but the period of active duty service excluding entry level and skill training is less than 18 months, the applicable active duty period is 18 months.

[65] Department of Veterans Affairs, "Post-9/11 G.I. Bill: Final Rule," 74 *Federal Register* 14659, March 31, 2009. Under the MGIB-AD, service members were allowed to contribute up to an additional $600 while on active duty in $20 monthly increments and receive up to an additional $5 monthly for each $20 contributed over the life of their entitlement period under what is known as the $600 Buy Up Program.

[66] The 15-year limitation does not include periods when an individual was ineligible for the program but their discharge status was later amended to make them eligible for the program, and periods when an individual was detained by a foreign government or power and any related recovery period in a hospital. Individuals incapable

of beginning education as a result of a physical or mental disability can be granted an extension for the period of incapacity.

[67] An "institution of higher learning" is an institution offering postsecondary level academic instruction that leads to an associate or higher degree if the school is empowered by the appropriate state education authority under state law to grant an associate or higher degree, or in the absence of a state education authority if the school is accredited for degree programs by a recognized accrediting agency. Institutions of higher learning are also hospitals offering educational programs at the postsecondary level and foreign educational institutions that offer courses leading to a standard college degree, or the equivalent, and which are recognized as such by the secretary of education (or a comparable official) of the country or other jurisdiction in which the institution is located. A standard college degree is an associate or higher degree awarded by (1) an IHL that is accredited as a collegiate institution by a recognized regional or national accrediting agency; (2) an IHL that is a "candidate" for accreditation as that term is used by the regional or national accrediting agencies; or (3) an IHL upon completion of a course which is accredited by an agency recognized to accredit specialized degree-level programs. An IHL is not the same as an institution of higher education (IHE) as defined in sections 101 and 102 of the Higher Education Act of 1965, as amended (HEA). An IHE admits as regular students only those who have a high school diploma or its equivalent or who are beyond the age of compulsory school attendance. Also, an IHE may be a less-than-two-year postsecondary vocational institutional or may provide one-year programs of education or training without having to provide an associate's or higher degree. With exceptions and the possibility of waivers, no more than 50% of an IHE's courses can be correspondence courses; no more than 50% of an IHE's students can be enrolled in correspondence courses; no more than 25% of the IHE's students may be incarcerated; and no more than 50% of an IHE's students may be without a high school diploma or its equivalent unless it offers an associate's or bachelor's degree. With exceptions, neither the IHE nor its affiliates can have filed for bankruptcy, and the IHE's owner or chief executive officer cannot have been guilty of a crime involving the acquisition, fraud, use, or expenditure of HEA Title IV funds. In addition, postsecondary institutions outside the United States must meet additional criteria to be considered IHEs.

[68] Although California's public colleges and universities only charge fees and do not charge resident undergraduate tuition, the VA and the California state approving agency reached an agreement to break up the fees into a tuition charge and fees charge for the purposes of the Post-9/11 GI Bill.

[69] U.S. Department of Veterans Affairs, 2009-10 Maximum In-State Tuition and Fees, available at http://www.gibill.va.gov/GI_Bill_Info/CH33/Tuition_and_fees.htm, last updated January 25, 2010.

[70] Tuition was reported to the U.S. Department of Education in the Integrated Postsecondary Education Data System (IPEDS).

[71] High fees are often related to flight training.

[72] U.S. Department of Veterans Affairs, 2009-10 Maximum In-State Tuition and Fees, available at http://www.gibill.va.gov/GI_Bill_Info/CH33/Tuition_and_fees.htm, last updated January 25, 2010.

[73] Distance education is defined in 20 U.S.C. § 1003(6) as education to deliver instruction to students who are separated from the instructor and to support regular and substantive interaction between the students and the instructor, synchronously or asynchronously, that uses one or more of the following technologies: the Internet; one- and two-way transmissions through open broadcast, closed circuit, cable, microwave, broadband lines, fiber optics, satellite, or wireless communications devices; audio conferencing; or video cassettes, DVDs, and CD-ROMs, if the cassettes, DVDs, or CD-ROMs are used in a course in conjunction with the Internet, one- and two-way transmissions, or audio conferencing.

[74] BAH is a DOD benefit to uniformed service members to provide housing compensation when government quarters are not provided. The amount is based on housing costs in local civilian housing markets and is payable based on geographic duty location, pay grade, and dependency status.

[75] U.S. Department of Defense, 2010 BAH Rates—WITH DEPENDENTS, available at http://www.defenstravel.dod.mil/pdc-archive/bah/acrobat/2010/FINAL%202010%20%27With%27%20Dependents%20BAH%20Rates.pdf as of December 16, 2009.

[76] The VA has determined in 38 CFR 2 1.9640 that a lump sum books and supplies stipend for each academic term equals $41.67 multiplied by the number of credit hours enrolled and multiplied by the ratio of the number of credit hours enrolled to the number of credit hours required for full-time pursuit.

[77] The entitlement period is reduced one month for each month enrolled.

[78] The entitlement period is reduced a fraction of a month for each month enrolled. The fraction is the ratio of the number of credit hours enrolled to the number of credit hours required for full-time pursuit of the degree program in which the student is enrolled.

[79] U.S. Department of Defense, *Directive-Type Memorandum (DTM) 09-003: Post 9/11 GI Bill*, June 22, 2009, p. 13, http://www.defenselink.mil/news/DTM%2009-003%20Post%209-11%20GI%20Bill%20Optimized1.pdf.

[80] Department of Veterans Affairs, "Post-9/11 GI Bill: Final Rule," 74 *Federal Register* 14656, 14689, March 31, 2009, clarifies the eligibility requirements for advance payments.

[81] This program is not related to the Yellow Ribbon Reintegration Program authorized by the National Defense Authorization Act for Fiscal Year 2008 (P.L. 110-181). The Yellow Ribbon Reintegration Program consists of informational events and activities for Reservists, their families, and community members to facilitate access

to services supporting their health and well-being through the pre-deployment, deployment, demobilization, and postdeployment-reconstitution.

[82] 38 CFR 21.9700 as of March 31, 2009.

[83] Tuition and fees were reported to the U.S. Department of Education in the Integrated Postsecondary Education Data System (IPEDS).

[84] Under the MGIB-AD, children are defined as unmarried persons under the age of 18, unmarried persons who became permanently incapable of self-support before the age of 18, or unmarried persons between the ages of 18 and 23 who are in school. Children must be legitimate children, acknowledged illegitimate children, legally adopted, or stepchildren who are members of the eligible individual's household.

[85] U.S. Department of Veterans Affairs, "Post-9/11 GI Bill: Marine Gunnery Sergeant John David Fry Scholarship," press release, http://www.gibill.va.gov/documents/Fry_Scholarship.pdf.

[86] U.S. Department of Defense, *Directive-Type Memorandum (DTM) 09-003: Post 9/11 GI Bill*, June 22, 2009, http://www.defenselink.mil/news/DTM%2009-003%20Post%209-1 1%20GI%20Bill%20Optimized1.pdf.

[87] Service members who become eligible for retirement on August 1, 2009, or who have an approved retirement date after August 1, 2009, and before July 1, 2010, are not required to serve additional time. Service members who become eligible for retirement after August 1, 2009, and before August 1, 2010, are required to serve one additional year of service. Service members who become eligible for retirement on or after August 1, 2010, and before August 1, 2011, are required to serve two additional years of service. Service members who become eligible for retirement on or after August 1, 2011, and before August 1, 2012, are required to serve three additional years of service.

[88] The transferred benefits could not be considered marital property in divorce proceedings.

[89] A service member is *delayed* if the person is listed as missing in action, captured in the line of duty, or forcibly detained as a result of active duty service

[90] A total permanent disability is any disability rated total for the purposes of disability compensation, which is based on an impairment reasonably certain to continue throughout the life of the disabled person.

[91] Children of Commonwealth Army veterans and New Philippine Scouts who meet the requirements of service-connected disability or death are also eligible.

[92] Under the MGIB-AD, children are defined as unmarried persons under the age of 18, unmarried persons who became permanently incapable of self-support before the age of 18, or unmarried persons between the ages of 18 and 23 who are in school. According to the authorizing language in 38 U.S.C. § 10 1(4), children must be legitimate children, acknowledged illegitimate children, legally adopted, or stepchildren who are members of the eligible individual's household.

[93] A spouse who is incapable of beginning education as a result of a physical or mental disability may be granted an extension of the 10-year entitlement period.

[94] There are allowable exceptions. The VA may make an exception for a child who is under 18 years of age and whose parent dies or has a total permanent disability as a result of a service-connected disability or has been delayed. The VA may allow eight years of eligibility to a child whose parent dies or has a total permanent disability as a result of a service-connected disability; may allow eight years of eligibility up to age 31 to a child whose parent has been delayed or after his/her own discharge or release from the armed forces; and may allow completion of a program of education suspended due to conditions beyond the child's control.

[95] Special restorative training is used to overcome, or lessen, the effects of a physical or mental disability that would handicap an eligible person in the pursuit of a program of education.

[96] The individual's entitlement period is reduced one month each time the collective amount paid is equal to $925.

[97] For apprentice or on-the-job training, an individual's entitlement period is reduced one month each time the collective amount paid is equal to the full-time institutional monthly benefit. Individuals working/training fewer than 120 hours monthly have their payment and entitlement period usage proportionately reduced.

[98] For licensing, certification, admissions, or course credit testing, an individual's entitlement period is reduced one month each time the collective amount paid is equal to the full-time institutional monthly benefit.

[99] Full-time training is determined by the capacities of the individual. Only full-time restorative training is eligible.

[100] An individual's entitlement period is reduced one day for each $30.83 in increase.

[101] 38 C.F.R. § 21.3023.

[102] Aggregate educational assistance may not exceed 48 months under the following programs: Parts VII or VIII, Veterans Regulation numbered 1(a), as amended; Title II of the Veterans' Readjustment Assistance Act of 1952; the War Orphans' Educational Assistance Act of 1956; Chapters 30, 32, 33, 34, 35, and 36 of Title 38 U.S.C. and the former chapter 33; Chapters 106a, 1606, and 1607 of Title 10 U.S.C.; section 903 of the Department of Defense Authorization Act, 1981 (10 U.S.C. 2141 note); the Hostage Relief Act of 1980 (5 U.S.C. 5561 note); and the Omnibus Diplomatic Security and Antiterrorism Act of 1986 (22 U.S.C. 4801). The VA may extend the aggregate entitlement period for educational assistance in combination with the vocational rehabilitation and employment program (Chapter 31 of Title 38).

[103] The value of $1,379 was calculated by CRS. It is the maximum amount of in-state required fees for full-time undergraduate students for the full academic year 2007-2008 for all 28 public two- and four-year colleges and universities in Colorado as reported in the U.S. Department of Education's Integrated Postsecondary Data

System under the variable labeled *IC2007_AY.FEE2:VL-In-state required fees for full-time undergraduates.* The fees represent the fixed sum charged to students for items not covered by tuition and required of such a large proportion of all students that the student who does not pay the charge is an exception.

[104] Elizabeth Redden, "GI Bill Lets Veterans Take Flight," *Inside Higher Ed*, July 10, 2009.

[105] For additional information, see CRS Report RL34627, *Veterans' Benefits: The Vocational Rehabilitation and Employment Program*, by Christine Scott and Carol D. Davis.

[106] The program of independent living services and assistance may be 24 months.

[107] 38 U.S.C. § 3108 et seq.

[108] The VA conducts disability evaluations and assigns disability ratings to service members and veterans. An individual's disability rating describes the impact of a disability on gainful employment in the civilian economy. The lower the rating, the more capable an individual is of maintaining gainful employment. For more information, see CRS Report RL33991, *Disability Evaluation of Military Servicemembers*, by Christine Scott and Don J. Jansen.

[109] Description prepared by CRS based on a historical review of legislation and other reports.

[110] The draft age was lowered from 20 to 18 years when President Roosevelt signed the Selective Service Act of 1942 (P.L. 77-772).

[111] Facts for Features, U.S. Census Bureau, April 29, 2004, http://www.census.gov/Press-Release/www/2004/cb04-ffse07.pdf.

[112] Historical National Population Estimates: July 1, 1900, to July 1, 1999, Source: Population Estimates Program, Population Division, U.S. Census Bureau, Internet Release Date: April 11, 2000, Revised date: June 28, 2000, http://www.census.gov/popest/archives/1990s/popclockest.txt.

[113] P.L. 79-268, enacted in 1945, removed the restriction limiting benefits beyond the first year to those whose education had been impaired, delayed, interrupted, or interfered with; those under 25 years of age; or those not pursuing refresher or retraining courses, thus opening the full program to all veterans.

[114] P.L. 85-807, enacted in 1958, extended benefits for veterans who through 1956 were ineligible for the program but whose discharge status was later amended to make them eligible for the program, allowing those veterans to begin a program of education within four years of the amended discharge status but before August 28, 1962, and allowing them no more than five years of benefits before January 31, 1965.

[115] U. S. Congress, House Committee on Veterans' Affairs, *Readjustment Benefits: General Survey and Appraisal, A Report on Veterans' Benefits in the United States*, committee print, prepared by The President's Commission on Veterans' Pensions, 84th Cong., 2nd sess., September 11, 1965, H.Prt. 289 (Washington: GPO, 1956), pp. 28-29.

[116] On-the-job training programs were required to gain approval from a state approving agency according to specific criteria under P.L. 79-679 enacted in 1946. Requirements for on-the-farm training programs were established in P.L. 80-377, enacted in 1947. With regard to vocational schools, P.L. 81-610, enacted in 1950, (1) authorized the VA to disapprove payment of benefits for training in for-profit vocational schools that had been in existence for less than one year, (2) prescribed stricter criteria for approval of for-profit schools with fewer than 25 students or one-fourth of the students enrolled (whichever was larger) paying their own tuition, (3) provided that no new courses could be approved in for-profit schools where the state approving agency determined that the occupation for which the course was intended to provide training was crowded in the state and that existing training facilities were adequate, and (4) set minimum attendance requirements for veterans pursuing trade or technical courses below college level.

[117] P.L. 80-262, enacted in 1949, and P.L. 81-266 and P.L. 81-610, enacted in 1950.

[118] The studies include a February 1950 joint report by the VA and the Bureau of the Budget, two reports issued in January 1951 and February 1952, by a House Select Committee to Investigate the Educational and Training Program under the GI Bill and a survey by the General Accounting Office of the education and training operations of the VA in seven states issued in July 1951.

[119] U.S. Congress, House Committee on Veterans' Affairs, *Readjustment Benefits: General Survey and Appraisal, A Report on Veterans' Benefits in the United States*, committee print, prepared by The President's Commission on Veterans' Pensions, 84th Cong., 2nd sess., September 11, 1965, H.Prt. 289 (Washington: GPO, 1956), p. 30.

[120] U.S. Congress, House Committee of the Whole House on the State of the Union, *Education and Other Benefits for Veterans of Service After January 31, 1955*, Report to accompany H.R. 12410, 89th Cong., 2nd sess., February 3, 1966, Report No. 1258, p. 3.

[121] U.S. Congress, House Committee on Veterans' Affairs, *Readjustment Benefits: Education and Training, and Employment and Unemployment, A Report on Veterans' Benefits in the United States*, committee print, prepared by The President's Commission on Veterans' Pensions, 84th Cong., 2nd sess., September 12, 1956, H.Prt. 291 (Washington: GPO, 1956), pp. 55-59.

[122] U.S. Congress, House Committee on Veterans' Affairs, *Readjustment Benefits: General Survey and Appraisal, A Report on Veterans' Benefits in the United States*, committee print, prepared by The President's Commission on Veterans' Pensions , 84th Cong., 2nd sess., September 11, 1965, H.Prt. 289 (Washington: GPO, 1956), p. 29.

[123] The 2008 inflation adjusted number for total expenditures was calculated by inflating $14.5 billion in 1956 dollars to 2008 using the U.S. Department of Labor's Bureau of Labor Statistics' Consumer Price Index-All Urban Consumers - (CPI-U) U.S. city average as reported at ftp://ftp.bls.gov/pub/special.requests/cpi/cpiai.txt.

[124] Description prepared by CRS based on a historical review of legislation and other reports.

[125] Historical National Population Estimates: July 1, 1900, to July 1, 1999, Source: Population Estimates Program, Population Division, U.S. Census Bureau, Internet Release Date: April 11, 2000, Revised date: June 28, 2000, http://www.census.gov/popest/archives/1990s/popclockest.txt.

[126] U.S. Congress, House Committee on Veterans' Affairs, *Readjustment Benefits: General Survey and Appraisal, A Report on Veterans' Benefits in the United States*, committee print, prepared by The President's Commission on Veterans' Pensions, 84th Cong., 2nd sess., September 11, 1965, H.Prt. 289 (Washington: GPO, 1956), p. 30.

[127] The January 31, 1955, termination date for eligibility was established by P.L. 84-7 enacted in 1955.

[128] P.L. 85-807 enacted in 1958 extended benefits for veterans who through 1956 were ineligible for the program but whose discharge status was later amended to make them eligible for the program allowing those veterans to begin a program of education within three years of the amended discharge status but before August 28, 1961, and allowing them no more than five years of benefits.

[129] The Attorney General's List of Subversive Organizations was prepared according to section three of part III of Executive Order 9835, which established a loyalty program to the federal government to thwart communism.

[130] U.S. Congress, House Committee on Veterans' Affairs, *Readjustment Benefits: General Survey and Appraisal, A Report on Veterans' Benefits in the United States*, committee print, prepared by The President's Commission on Veterans' Pensions, 84th Cong., 2nd sess., September 11, 1965, H.Prt. 289 (Washington: GPO, 1956), pp. 28-31, 153- 154.

[131] Starr, Paul, *The Discarded Army*, p. 237.

[132] U. S. Congress, House Committee on Veterans' Affairs, *Readjustment Benefits: General Survey and Appraisal, A Report on Veterans' Benefits in the United States*, committee print, prepared by The President's Commission on Veterans' Pensions, 84th Cong., 2nd sess., September 11, 1965, H.Prt. 289 (Washington: GPO, 1956), pp. 37-40.

[133] U.S. Congress, House Committee on Veterans' Affairs, *Readjustment Benefits: General Survey and Appraisal, A Report on Veterans' Benefits in the United States*, committee print, prepared by The President's Commission on Veterans' Pensions, 84th Cong., 2nd sess., September 11, 1965, H.Prt. 289 (Washington: GPO, 1956), p.154.

[134] U.S. Congress, House Committee on Veterans' Affairs, *Readjustment Benefits: General Survey and Appraisal, A Report on Veterans' Benefits in the United States*, committee print, prepared by The President's Commission on Veterans' Pensions, 84th Cong., 2nd sess., September 11, 1965, H.Prt. 289 (Washington: GPO, 1956), p. 30.

[135] Veterans pursuing programs of education that combined flight training and other coursework could be reimbursed for 75% of the cost of flight training and receive a monthly allowance. Their entitlement period was reduced at a rate of one day for every $1.25 in payments.

[136] Description prepared by CRS based on a historical review of legislation and other reports.

[137] By presidential proclamation, the Vietnam Era began on February 28, 1961, and terminated on May 7, 1975, for veterans who served in the Republic of Vietnam during that period, and the Vietnam Era began on August 5, 1964, and ended on May 7, 1975, in all other cases.

[138] John T. Woolley and Gerhard Peters, *The American Presidency Project* [online], Santa Barbara, CA: University of California (hosted), Gerhard Peters (database). http://www.presidency

[139] U.S. Congress, Senate Committee on Labor and Public Welfare, Cold War Veterans' Readjustment Assistance Act; report to accompany S. 9. Senate Report No. 89-269, 89th Congress, 1st Session, (Washington: GPO, 1965), p. 15.

[140] U.S. Congress, Senate Committee on Labor and Public Welfare, Subcommittee on Veterans' Affairs, *Cold War GI Bill - 1965*, S. 9: A Bill to Provide Readjustment Assistance to Veterans who Serve in the Armed Forces During the Induction Period, 89th Cong., 1st sess., February 8, 18, 19, 24, 26, March 1, 9, 1965, (Washington: GPO, 1965), pp. 66- 67.

[141] Veterans who were ineligible for the program on discharge or release but whose discharge status was later amended to make them eligible for the program were allowed benefits for up to eight years (later extended to 10 years by P.L. 93-337, enacted in 1974) after the discharge status was amended. Veterans who were incapable of beginning education as a result of a physical or mental disability could be granted an extension for the period of incapacity according to P.L. 95-202, enacted in 1977. P.L. 97-72, enacted in 1981, authorized the VA to provide educational assistance through December 31, 1983, to Vietnam Era veterans whose 10-year delimiting date had expired but who had remaining dollars of entitlement and entitlement period, if the extended eligibility were used for apprentice or on-the-job training, a program with a vocational objective, or a program of secondary education, and if the VA determined that the veteran was in need of such a program to achieve a suitable occupational or vocational objective.

[142] Veterans were allowed one change of their educational objective if not making satisfactory progress (by no fault of misconduct, neglect, or lack of application) and allowed one additional change if the new program fit their aptitude or if there was a reduced likelihood of not making satisfactory progress as a result of their own misconduct, neglect, or lack of application.

[143] P.L. 91-219, enacted in 1970, added provisions allowing the disapproval of bartending, personal development, and sales courses, which do not provide specialized training in a specific vocation. P.L. 96-466, enacted in 1980, further clarified that over the preceding two years at least 50% of the graduates of vocational programs of education who were available for employment had to be employed in that vocational area for an average of 10 hours weekly for the educational program to gain approval. This provision was repealed by P.L. 97-306, enacted in 1982, because it was determined to no longer be necessary to prevent abuse.

[144] Eligible individuals include veterans, service members, and surviving spouses and children eligible to receive benefits under the War Orphans Educational Assistance Program (Title 38 U.S.C., Chapter 35).

[145] Full-time attendance required a minimum of 30 hours per week for trade or technical courses below college level involving mostly shop practice, required a minimum of 25 hours per week for institutional courses below college level involving mostly theoretical classroom instruction, required a minimum of four units per year for academic high school courses, required a minimum of 14 credit hours (or less if certified by the institution according to P.L. 91-219, enacted in 1970) for institutional undergraduate courses, and required a 30-hour work week or the minimum established by the training establishment for apprentice and on-the-job training according to P.L. 9 1-584, enacted in 1970.

[146] P.L. 90-77, enacted in 1967, provided a payment schedule based on the first through fourth and succeeding six month periods of full-time apprentice or on-the-job training and the number of dependents. The maximum monthly payment was up to $100 monthly for the first six months of training if the student had two or more dependents (eventually increased to $336 by P.L. 98-543, enacted in 1984). P.L. 90-77 also allowed cooperative farm trainees $80 per month (eventually increased to up to $404 monthly for two dependents based on full-, three-quarter- and half-time status and the number of dependents by P.L. 98-543, enacted in 1984).

[147] P.L. 91-219, enacted in 1970, created the PREP, and P.L. 94-502, enacted in 1976, terminated the PREP.

[148] Description prepared by CRS based on a historical review of legislation and other reports.

[149] The exceptions to the September 30, 1981, end date were Vietnam Era veterans who were continuing full-time training in the first two years following the expiration of their entitlement period or who were already pursuing flight training courses when flight training benefits were eliminated.

[150] U.S. General Accounting Office, *Veterans Administration Education Loan Program Should Be Terminated: Legislative Action Taken*, HRD-81-128, August 28, 1981, http://archive.gao.gov/f0102/116325.pdf.

In: Veterans Benefits
Editors: George B. Meyers and Alice M. Glaskin
ISBN: 978-1-61209-581-3

Chapter 11

VETERANS' BENEFITS: PENSION BENEFIT PROGRAM

Christine Scott and Carol D. Davis

SUMMARY

The Department of Veterans Affairs (VA) administers several pension benefit programs for veterans as well as their surviving spouses and dependent children. The most current pension programs available (for those meeting the eligibility criteria on or after January 1, 1979) are the Improved Disability Pension for certain low-income veterans and the Improved Death Pension for certain low-income surviving spouses or children of veterans. There is also a special pension for Medal of Honor recipients. This chapter describes these programs, including the eligibility criteria and current benefit levels.

OVERVIEW

The Department of Veterans Affairs (VA) administers several pension programs for veterans and their surviving spouses and dependent children. There are two types of pension programs administered by the VA: (1) pension programs for veterans of specific periods of war; and (2) pension programs for certain low-income veterans. The pension programs for specific periods of war are for periods before World War I. They include pension programs for veterans, as well as their surviving spouses and dependent children, of certain periods of war such as the Civil War, the Indian Wars, and the Spanish-American War. The pension programs for certain low-income veterans include the Old Law Disability Pension, the Section 306 Disability Pension, and the Improved Disability Pension. The VA pension programs for certain low-income surviving spouses and dependent children of veterans include the Old Law Death Pension, the Section 306 Death Pension, and the Improved Death Pension.

In addition to the pension programs related to periods of service for certain low-income veterans and surviving spouses and dependent children, the VA administers a special pension program for Medal of Honor recipients.

This chapter will provide information on the most current pension programs—those programs for which a veteran, a surviving spouse, or a dependent child becomes eligible on or after January 1, 1 979—and on the special pension program for Medal of Honor recipients. The current pension program for veterans is the Improved Disability Pension, which is for certain low-income veterans. The current pension program for certain low-income surviving spouses and dependent children of veterans is the Improved Death Pension. Both pension programs were created by P.L. 95-588, the Veterans and Survivors Pension Improvement Act of 1978.

The Improved Disability Pension Benefit

The Improved Disability Pension provides a monthly benefit to certain low-income veterans. The monthly benefit is based on a maximum annual benefit, and the actual benefit received by the veteran reflects a reduction (from the maximum amount) of the veteran's "countable" income. This means that a veteran with countable income above the maximum benefit amount is not eligible for the pension.

Maximum Annual Benefit Amount

The maximum annual benefit amounts for the veterans' pension benefit are set in statute[1] and are based on the presence of a spouse or dependent child (or children) and the need for aid and attendance.[2] The annual benefit amounts are adjusted automatically by law[3] each year to reflect a cost-of-living adjustment (COLA) equal to the COLA for Social Security benefits. For example, beginning December 1, 2008, the maximum annual amount for the pension benefit in 2009 and 2010 is $11,830 for a veteran and $15,493 for a veteran with one dependent.[4] If two veterans are married to each other, the maximum annual amount is $15,493, the same as for a veteran with one dependent. The maximum annual benefit amount will be higher if the veteran is housebound or requires aid and attendance.[5]

Eligibility Criteria

To be eligible for the pension benefit, a veteran must meet eligibility criteria related to combat/period of service; income/net worth; and age or disability.

Combat/Period of Service

A veteran must meet military service requirements related to combat, or service during a period of war to be eligible for the pension benefit.[6] Specifically, a veteran must have been discharged from military service under conditions other than dishonorable and must have served in the active military:

- for at least 90 days during a period of war;[7]
- during a period of war and was released from service for a service-connected disability;
- for 90 or more consecutive days which began or ended during a period of war; or
- for a total of 90 days or more in two or more separate periods of service during one or more periods of war.

Income/Net Worth

As noted previously, the pension benefit for a veteran who meets the other eligibility requirements (combat/period of service and disability/age) is calculated by subtracting the veteran's annual countable income from the statutory annual maximum benefit. This means that a veteran with annual countable income above the annual maximum benefit amount will receive no pension benefit. A veteran with annual countable income below the annual maximum benefit amount will have his or her benefit reduced dollar for dollar by the amount of annual countable income. In addition, a veteran may not have a net worth, or estate, large enough that it would be reasonable for part of the estate to be used for the veteran's maintenance.[8]

Annual countable income includes income from nearly all sources. However, there are several specific sources of income that are *not included* in determining annual countable income:[9]

- donations from public welfare or private relief organizations;
- pension benefits administered by the VA;
- expenses paid by a veteran's spouse (or the veteran's surviving spouse or child) for the veteran's last illness, burial, or debts;
- amounts paid by the veteran for the last illness and burial of the veteran's spouse or child;
- amounts paid by a veteran's spouse for the last illness and burial of the veteran's child;
- insurance reimbursement for property casualty loss (up to the greater of fair market value or replacement value);
- profit from disposing of personal or real property (other than in the course of business);
- amounts in joint accounts the veteran acquires by the death of the other owner(s);
- amounts paid by the veteran, spouse, or child for unreimbursed medical expenses (limited to the excess above 5% of the pension benefit);
- up to $5,000 paid as a veteran's benefit due to injury or disease by a state or municipality (for determinations of income for calendar years beginning after October 1, 2011);[10] and
- amounts paid by a veteran or surviving spouse to pursue education, vocational rehabilitation, or training, including tuition, fees, books, and, if the veteran or surviving spouse needs aid and attendance, travel expenses above reasonable expenses for a nondisabled person.

Disability/Age

To be eligible for the pension benefit, the veteran must be totally disabled[11] due to non-service connected injuries or illnesses that are not a result of the veteran's willful misconduct.[12] However, to determine if a veteran is totally disabled, the Secretary of Veterans Affairs may combine the disability ratings for service-connected disabilities with the disability ratings for non-service connected disabilities. The restriction is that if the veteran's service-connected disabilities have contributed to making the veteran eligible for the pension benefit, the veteran will receive the greater of the pension benefit or the disability compensation benefit (for the service-connected disabilities). A veteran cannot receive both disability compensation and the pension benefit.

P.L. 107-103, the Veterans Education and Benefit Expansion Act of 2001, extended the pension benefit to veterans aged 65 or over, regardless of disability status (or disability rating), who meet the other pension requirements (combat/period and income/net worth).

Other

The pension benefit for a veteran convicted of a felony or misdemeanor will be stopped beginning 61 days after the veteran is imprisoned, and it will resume when the imprisonment ends. The veteran's pension benefit may be paid to the veteran's spouse or dependent children during the veteran's imprisonment.

To apply for the pension benefit, a veteran must complete and submit VA Form 21-526, which is the application form for both disability compensation and the pension benefit. As part of the claims processing, the veteran will receive a disability rating, which may require a physical examination.

Interaction with Social Security and Supplemental Security Income (SSI)

Countable income for the veterans' pension benefit includes any Social Security benefits received. Therefore, the receipt of Social Security benefits can reduce or eliminate a veteran's pension benefit. Countable income does not include any Supplemental Security Income (S SI) payments received. However, because the SSI program includes veterans' benefits as unearned income in calculating the income limitations for SSI, a veteran's pension benefit could reduce the veteran's SSI benefit.[13]

THE IMPROVED DEATH PENSION BENEFIT

The surviving spouse or dependent child of a veteran may be eligible for the Improved Death Pension Benefit if eligibility requirements with respect to the deceased veteran and surviving spouse or dependent child are met, along with an income requirement.

Deceased Veteran

The deceased veteran must have met the military service requirements for the Improved Disability Pension with respect to the veteran's discharge and period of service.[14] However, for the Improved Death Pension, an individual who has at least two years of honorable military service and who dies in military service but not in the line of duty is also considered a veteran.[15]

Surviving Spouse

The surviving spouse cannot be remarried and must have been married to the deceased veteran:[16]

- for at least one year (there is no minimum if the surviving spouse and veteran had a child), and
- must have been wed before December 14, 1944 for deceased veterans of the Mexican border period and World War I; before January 1, 1957 for deceased veterans of World War II; before February 1, 1965 for deceased veterans of the Korean conflict; before May 8, 1985 for deceased veterans of the Vietnam era; or before January 1, 2001 for deceased veterans of the Persian Gulf War.

Surviving Children

Surviving children must be under age 18 (or under age 23 if in school) or must have become incapable of self-care before age 18.

Income

The countable income for a surviving spouse or child is calculated like that of a veteran for the Improved Disability Pension. However, for a surviving spouse with custody of a deceased veteran's child, part of the child's income that is available to the surviving spouse may be included in countable income. [17] For a veteran's surviving child, his or her current work income is excluded from countable income, if the income is not more than the income level at which a federal income tax return must be filed[18] *plus* postsecondary education or vocational rehabilitation or training expenses paid by the child.[19] In addition, for a surviving spouse or child, the proceeds from a life insurance policy on the veteran is excluded from countable income.[20]

Maximum Benefit Amount

The maximum annual benefit amounts for surviving spouses and dependent children, like those for veterans, are set in statute and are automatically increased to reflect the COLA for Social Security benefits. For example, effective December 1, 2008,[21] the maximum annual benefit amounts in 2009 and 2010 for a surviving spouse without a dependent child is $7,933, and $10,385 for a surviving spouse with a dependent child (there is an incremental amount for each dependent child). Maximum annual benefit amounts are higher if the surviving spouse is housebound or requires aid and attendance.[22] For a surviving child, the maximum annual benefit amount is $2,020.

MEDAL OF HONOR PENSION

A veteran who has been awarded a Medal of Honor is eligible for a monthly pension ($1,194 as of December 1, 2008, for 2009 and 201 0).[23] Eligibility for the pension is based solely on receipt of the Medal of Honor, and receipt of the special pension (the Medal of Honor recipient must elect to receive the special pension) does not reduce any other benefits under U.S. law. A veteran who has received more than one Medal of Honor is, however, limited to receiving only one Medal of Honor pension benefit.[24]

End Notes

[1] 38 U.S.C. §1521(b)-§1521(g).

[2] Aid and attendance is provided when a veteran needs another person's help to perform activities of daily living, such as eating, dressing, or taking a shower.

[3] 38 U.S.C. §53 12.

[4] For more information on the Social Security COLA, see CRS Report 94-803, *Social Security: Cost-of-Living Adjustments*, by Gary Sidor.

[5] For more information on current rates, please see the Department of Veterans Affairs website at http://www.vba.va.gov/bln/21/Rates/pen01.htm.

[6] 38 U.S.C. §1521(j).

[7] For information on periods of war, see CRS Report RS2 1405, *U.S. Periods of War*, by Barbara Salazar Torreon.

[8] 38 U.S.C. § 1522.

[9] 38 U.S.C. §1503.

[10] Provision was part of the Veterans' Benefits Act of 2010 (P.L. 111-275).

[11] The VA rates disability on a scale of 0-100 in 10% increments, with 100% being totally disabled. The rating is used for pensions and for disability compensation. For more information on disability evaluation by the VA, see the "VA Disability Evaluation" section of CRS Report RL33991, *Disability Evaluation of Military Servicemembers*, by Christine Scott and Don J. Jansen.

[12] 38 U.S.C. §1513 and 38 U.S.C. §1521.

[13] For more information on the SSI program, see CRS Report 94-486, *Supplemental Security Income (SSI): A Fact Sheet*, by Scott Szymendera, and CRS Report RS20294, *SSI Income and Resource Limits: A Fact Sheet*, by Scott Szymendera.

[14] 38 U.S.C. §1541(a) and §1542(a).

[15] 38 U.S.C. §1541(h).

[16] 38 U.S.C. §1541(f).

[17] 38 U.S.C. §1541(g).

[18] The income level at which a tax return must be filed (the filing requirement) is equal to the sum of the standard deduction and personal exemption amounts. For tax year 2009, the filing requirement for a single taxpayer is $9,350 for a taxpayer under age 65.

[19] 38 U.S.C. §1503(a)(10).

[20] 38 U.S.C. §1503(a)(11).

[21] These For more information on the Social Security COLA, see CRS Report 94-803, *Social Security: Cost-of-Living Adjustments*, by Gary Sidor

[22] For more information on current rates, please see the Department of Veterans Affairs website at http://www.vba.va.gov/bln/21/Rates/pen02.htm.

[23] The pension benefit was increased to $1,000 and a COLA was provided by P.L. 107-3 30, the Veterans Benefits Act of 2002.

[24] 38 U.S.C. §1562.

In: Veterans Benefits
Editors: George B. Meyers and Alice M. Glaskin ISBN: 978-1-61209-581-3

Chapter 12

VETERAN' BENEFITS: BURIAL BENEFITS AND NATIONAL CEMETERIES

Christine Scott

SUMMARY

Burial benefits are monetary and nonmonetary benefits that eligible veterans receive for their military service. Nonmonetary burial benefits have been provided to servicemembers and veterans since the Civil War. Monetary burial benefits have been provided to servicemembers and veterans since World War I.

Eligible veterans and active duty members of the Armed Forces can be interred in national cemeteries and can receive government-furnished headstones or markers, presidential memorial certificates, and burial flags. Their spouses or surviving spouses, minor children, and, under certain conditions, unmarried adult children may also be buried in national cemeteries.

Department of Veterans Affairs (VA) burial allowances are partial reimbursements for eligible veterans' burial and funeral costs. The allowance amount provided depends on whether the veteran's cause of death was service-connected or non-service-connected, or whether the death occurred in a VA facility. The next of kin to the veteran is eligible for reimbursement if he or she paid for the veteran's burial or funeral and has not been reimbursed by another government agency or some other source, such as the deceased veteran's employer.

The development of national cemeteries began as a result of the increasing number of Civil War casualties. The National Cemetery Act of 1867 was the first major piece of legislation to provide funds for, and directives about, national cemeteries. Today, there are 131 national cemeteries, along with 33 soldier's lots and monument sites, under the jurisdiction of the VA.

Several bills have been introduced in the 111th Congress that would affect nonmonetary and monetary benefits, and national cemeteries: H.R. 174, H.R. 217, H.R. 731, H.R. 1037,

H.R. 1114, H.R. 1163, H.R. 2586, H.R. 2594, H.R. 2642, H.R. 3544, H.R. 3949, H.R. 4044, H.R. 4045, H.R. 5879, H.R. 6042, S. 691, S. 728, and S. 746.

This chapter provides a descriptive analysis of both nonmonetary and monetary burial benefits and national cemeteries. It addresses congressional and constituent issues, such as who is eligible to receive burial benefits; who can be buried in a national cemetery; what plans does the VA have to build new or expand existing national cemeteries; and what benefits does the VA provide, among others. These issues may be of particular interest to Congress due to the aging of the veteran population, the changes to eligibility requirements, and recent VA report findings and recommendations related to the establishment of national cemeteries.

INTRODUCTION

The Department of Veterans Affairs (VA) provides a range of benefits and services to veterans who meet certain eligibility rules; benefits include hospital and medical care, disability compensation and pensions,[1] education,[2] vocational rehabilitation and employment services,[3] assistance to homeless veterans,[4] home loan guarantees,[5] administration of life insurance as well as traumatic injury protection insurance for servicemembers, and death benefits that cover burial expenses.

The department carries out its programs nationwide through three administrations and the Board of Veterans Appeals (BVA). The Veterans Health Administration (VHA) is responsible for health care services and medical and prosthetic research programs. The Veterans Benefits Administration (VBA) is responsible for, among other things, providing compensation, pensions, and education assistance. The National Cemetery Administration (NCA)[6] is responsible for maintaining national veterans cemeteries; providing grants to states for establishing, expanding, or improving state veterans cemeteries; and providing headstones and markers for the graves of eligible persons, among other things.

Burial benefits are monetary and nonmonetary benefits that eligible veterans receive for their service in the Armed Forces. As time progresses, the size of national cemeteries and the burial benefits program have increased.

Veterans or active duty servicemembers eligible for nonmonetary burial benefits can be interred in national cemeteries and can receive government-furnished headstones or markers, presidential memorial certificates, and burial flags. Their spouses or surviving spouses, minor children, and, under certain conditions, unmarried adult children may also be buried in national cemeteries.

Monetary burial benefits are partial reimbursements that the next of kin of eligible veterans can receive for burial and funeral costs.[7] The amount of the reimbursement depends on whether the veteran's cause of death was service-connected or non-service-connected, or whether the death occurred in a VA facility.[8]

National cemeteries, beginning as a result of Civil War casualties, have expanded to include 131 cemeteries, as well as 33 soldier's lots and monument sites, under the jurisdiction of the Department of Veterans Affairs.[9]

This chapter focuses on burial benefits provided by the VA. It does not discuss national cemeteries under the National Park Service, national cemeteries under the jurisdiction of the

American Battle Monument Commission, or Arlington National Cemetery, which is within the jurisdiction of the Department of the Army.

VETERANS' BURIAL BENEFITS

Eligibility Requirements for Burial in a National Cemetery

Under current federal regulation, the following persons are eligible for burial in a VA national cemetery:[10]

- Any member of the Armed Forces of the United States who dies while on active duty;
- Veterans who are discharged under conditions other than dishonorable (with certain exceptions);[11]
- U.S. citizens who may have served in the armed forces of a U.S. ally during a time of war (service must have been terminated honorably by death or otherwise);
- Members of Reserve Components and the Reserve Officer Training Corps (ROTC);
- Commissioned officers of the National Oceanic and Atmospheric Administration;
- Commissioned officers of the Regular or Reserve Corps of the U.S. Public Health Service;
- World War II merchant mariners;
- Any Filipino veteran who was a U.S. citizen or an alien lawfully admitted for permanent residence who was residing in the United States at the time of his or her death;
- The spouse or surviving spouse of an eligible veteran; and
- Minor and unmarried adult children of an eligible veteran.[12]

The Veterans' Benefits Act of 2010 (P.L. 111-275) provided that a natural or adoptive parent of an interred person who died from a training-related injury or was a hostile casualty,[13] would be eligible for burial in a national cemetery if (1) it is determined that there is space at the gravesite of the interred person; and (2) the interred person at the time of death did not have a spouse, surviving spouse, or child who is buried, or eligible to be buried, in a national cemetery.[14] All other persons seeking interment in a national cemetery must be approved by the Secretary of Veterans Affairs.[15]

The VA does not provide cremation or funeral arrangement services, which must be made through private funeral providers or cremation offices. The Department of Defense under the National Defense Authorization Act for FY2000 (P.L. 106-65) does provide, at the request of the family, a military honors ceremony that includes folding and presenting the U.S. burial flag and playing of "Taps."

Ineligible Persons

According to the VA website, persons who are not eligible for burial in a VA national cemetery are[16]

- former spouses of eligible individuals whose marriages to those individuals were terminated by annulment or divorce, if not otherwise eligible;
- family members other than those specified as eligible above;
- persons whose separation from the Armed Forces was under dishonorable conditions or whose character of service resulted in a bar to veterans' benefits;
- a person who was ordered to report to an induction station but was not actually inducted into military service;
- a person convicted of a federal or state capital crime, for which a sentence of imprisonment for life or the death penalty may be imposed and the conviction is final;[17]
- any person convicted of subversive activities after September 1, 1959;
- persons whose only service is active duty for training or inactive duty training in the National Guard or Reserve Component, unless the individual meets the eligibility criteria listed above; or
- members of groups whose service has been determined by the Secretary of the Air Force under the provisions of Title IV of the GI Bill Improvements Act (P.L. 95-202) as not warranting entitlement to benefits administered by the VA.

Nonmonetary Burial Benefits

Eligible veterans and active duty members of the Armed Forces can be interred in a national cemetery and receive a government-furnished headstone or marker, a presidential memorial certificate, and a burial flag.

Headstones, Markers, and Private Cemetery Medallions

All veterans who were discharged for reasons other than dishonorable and whose deaths occurred on or after November 1, 1990, are eligible to receive government-furnished headstones or markers.[18] The VA only furnishes headstones or markers to veterans whose deaths occurred before November 1, 1990, if the graves are not marked with private headstones. Spouses and other eligible dependents of veterans are eligible for headstones or markers only if they are interred in national, military post/base, or state cemeteries.

Veterans or members of their families have the option of selecting flat bronze, granite, or marble markers, or upright granite or marble headstones. However, the chosen style must be consistent with existing monuments at the place of burial.[19] Under current federal regulation, individuals who served in the Armed Forces after September 7, 1980, must have served a minimum of 24 consecutive months on active duty to be eligible for this benefit. Exceptions can be made to this rule by the Secretary under certain circumstances (e.g., death while on active duty). Only the next of kin may apply for a headstone, a marker, or a medallion.[20]

Memorial headstones, markers, and medallions are available for individual veterans or groups of veterans including those who die while on active duty whose remains are not recovered or are unidentified, have remains buried at sea, have remains donated to science, or whose cremated remains have been scattered. Spouses and dependents whose remains are unavailable for interment may also be furnished with memorial headstones in national, military post/base, or state cemeteries. This service is not available for spouses and dependents who are buried in private cemeteries. The application for a government-furnished headstone or marker can be found on the VA website.[21]

Veterans whose deaths occurred on or after November 1, 1990, and are buried in privately marked graves in private cemeteries may elect to receive medallions instead of government-furnished headstones or markers. The medallion, which represents the status of the deceased as a veteran, may be furnished at the request of the veteran's next of kin. The veteran cannot receive both a medallion and a government-furnished headstone or marker.

Regardless of the date of death, the VA will furnish the unmarked grave of a veteran, in any cemetery anywhere in the world, with a government headstone or marker.

Inscriptions

Government-furnished headstones and markers must be inscribed with the legal name of the deceased, branch of service, and the year of birth and death, in this order. Memorial markers must also include *"In Memory Of"* at the top. If space is available, the inscription may also contain any or all of the following: veteran's rank, war service, military decorations, awards, and month and day of birth and death. All of these elements must be inscribed in the English language.

Additions to the legal name, such as Doctor or Reverend, are not permitted on the mandatory name line of the headstone or marker. However, terms of endearment, nicknames, and other additional personalized inscriptions may, if space is available, be added at the bottom of the headstone or marker with the approval of the VA, which will determine if the requested inscription is judged to be respectful and in good taste.

Headstones and markers may also include emblems of belief, if so desired by the veteran or next of kin. According to the Code of Federal Regulations (CFR), an emblem of belief is "an emblem that represents the decedent's religious affiliation or sincerely held religious belief system, or a sincerely held belief system that was functionally equivalent to a religious belief system in the life of the decedent."[22] The VA maintains a list of approved emblems of belief.[23]

Presidential Memorial Certificates

The Presidential Memorial Certificate (PMC) program was initiated in March 1962 by President John F. Kennedy and has been continued by all subsequent Presidents. The PMC is a gold embossed paper certificate inscribed with the veteran's name that bears the President's signature. It honors the memory of honorably discharged deceased veterans.[24] The application for the PMC can be found on the VA website.[25]

In August 2008, the Department of Veterans Affairs released its *Evaluation of the VA Burial Benefits Program: Final Report*. The report conducted surveys and focus groups of veterans and their families. Of the aforementioned benefits, receiving a burial flag, a government-furnished headstone or marker, and military honors at the funeral service are benefits that are widely known by veterans and their families. However, the PMC is not as well known as the other benefits.

According to the report, "Of the 37 veteran next of kin participants, only one knew about the Presidential Memorial Certificate (PMC) benefit. Of 29 funeral directors, only two knew about the PMC benefit." The report also stated that "five out of every six veterans had never heard of the PMC."[26]

The report made the following two major recommendations related to the PMC:[27]

- "Conduct an outreach campaign to better promote the PMC among veterans, veteran family members, and funeral directors";
- "Develop an Internet Web-based tool so that next of kin and friends can apply online for a PMC, which would raise the visibility and value of the PMC. Creating this application is an investment for the future, as the demographics of the veteran population changes to comprise more of those who are comfortable with the Web."

Burial Flag

The VA will provide a free U.S. flag to the next of kin to drape the casket or accompany the urn of a deceased veteran who served honorably in the U.S. Armed Forces. Like the PMC, it is provided to honor the memory of a veteran's military service to his or her country. Generally, the flag is given to the next of kin at the funeral service as a keepsake. The family may donate the flag to a national cemetery with an Avenue of Flags to be flown on patriotic holidays.[28] The VA will furnish a burial flag to memorialize the following veterans who were discharged under other than dishonorable conditions:[29]

- veterans who served during wartime;
- veterans who died while on active duty after May 27, 1941;
- veterans who served after January 31, 1955;
- peacetime veterans who were discharged or released before June 27, 1950;
- certain persons who served in the organized military forces of the Commonwealth of the Philippines while in service of the U.S. Armed Forces and who died on or after April 25, 1951; and
- certain former members of the Selected Reserves.

Generally, the funeral director assists the next of kin in applying for a burial flag. However, the application can also be found on the VA website.[30]

Monetary Burial Benefits[31]

The VA burial allowances are partial reimbursements for the burial and funeral costs of eligible veterans and are not intended to cover the full burial or funeral costs. The allowance amount provided depends on whether the veteran's cause of death was service-connected, non-service-connected, or occurred in a VA facility.

Eligibility

The next of kin to the veteran is eligible for reimbursement if he or she paid for the veteran's burial or funeral and has not been reimbursed by another government agency or some other source, such as the deceased veteran's employer.[32]

Veteran Requirements

In addition to the above next of kin requirements, the deceased veteran must have been discharged under conditions other than dishonorable and met at least one of the following requirements:

- died because of a service-connected disability;
- was receiving a VA pension or compensation at the time of death;
- was eligible to receive a VA pension or compensation, but decided not to so as to avoid a reduction in his or her military retirement or disability pay;
- died while hospitalized at a VA facility, or while receiving care under VA contract at a non-VA facility;
- died while traveling under proper authorization and at VA expense to or from a specified place for the purpose of medical examination, treatment, or care;
- had an original or reopened claim pending at the time of death and had been found to be entitled to compensation or pension from a date prior to the date of death; or
- died on or after October 9, 1996, while a patient at a VA-approved state nursing home.

Burial and Plot-Interment Allowance Amount

Non-Service-Connected Deaths

The VA is authorized to pay up to $300 toward a veteran's funeral and burial expenses and up to $300 toward plot-interment costs.[33] These allowances are only for veterans whose deaths occurred on or after December 1, 2001. For veterans whose deaths occurred before December 1, 2001, there is a plot-interment allowance of $150. The Veterans' Benefits Act of 2010 (P.L. 111-275) increases the plot allowance to $700 for deaths occurring after September 30, 2011, and provides for an inflation adjustment of the plot allowance beginning in FY2013.

A veteran's net assets at the time of death do not affect the amount of burial allowance that the next of kin can receive. However, the allowance will be reduced if the burial expenses are paid by the veteran's employer, state, or another government source.[34] In either case, the burial allowance is limited to the difference between the amount the veteran's employer or another government source pays and the maximum amount the Secretary of VA may reimburse. No burial allowances are paid to public or private organizations.[35]

Death in a VA Facility

If the death of a veteran occurred while he or she was in a VA hospital, under VA-contracted nursing home care, or under nursing home care in which payments were being made by the VA (e.g., in a state nursing home), the Secretary of VA will pay the veteran's burial and funeral costs, not to exceed $300. In addition, some or all of the costs for transporting the veteran's remains to the state in which he or she will be interred may be reimbursed. However, the VA does not reimburse the costs for transporting the remains of veterans whose deaths occur in other countries.[36]

Service-Connected Deaths

The VA must pay up to $2,000 of the veteran's funeral and burial expenses if the veteran died as a result of a service-connected disability.[37] If the veteran's death occurred prior to September 10, 2001, the VA will pay up to $1,500 of the funeral and burial expenses. If the veteran is buried in a national cemetery, some or all of the cost for transporting the veteran's remains may be reimbursed.

2008 Report Findings and Recommendations

After examining the non-service-connected and service-connected burial and plot allowances, the aforementioned VA report found that the allowances were not meeting their original intent. According to the report, "the intent of the burial and plot allowances are to provide financial assistance to be used on behalf of veterans to offset their burial, funeral and plot costs."[38] Funeral costs have increased at a rate greater than that of other prices since 1990. While recognizing that it is not the intent of the Secretary of VA to cover the cost of the veteran's entire funeral and burial, it concludes that "significant increases in the allowances are necessary to restore the value of these important benefits to original levels."[39] Adjustments have been made to the allowances since 1973 (the first year of service-connected burial allowances), but they have not kept up with the inflation of funeral and burial expenses. According to the report, in 1973, the service-connected burial allowance, non-service-connected burial allowance and plot allowance were found to be 72% of service-connected funeral and burial costs, 22% of non-service-connected funeral and burial costs and 54% of burial plot costs, respectively. By 2007, the value of these allowances had decreased significantly, representing 23% of service-connected funeral and burial costs, 4% of non-service-connected funeral and burial costs and 14% of burial plot costs, respectively.[40]

The report made the following two major recommendations:

- Establish a basis for each allowance, which should be a percentage of the average cost of a funeral, burial, and burial plot. As outlined above, these percentages were estimated to be the following in 1973:
  - Service-connected allowance—72% of funeral and burial costs;
  - Non-service-connected allowance—22% of funeral and burial costs; and
  - Plot allowance—54% of burial plot costs.
- "Develop an annual schedule for reviewing and adjusting the allowances for funeral, burial, and burial plot costs using the Consumer Price Index for funeral expenses maintained by the Bureau of Labor Statistics."[41]

NATIONAL CEMETERIES

The History of National Cemeteries[42]

The development of national cemeteries began as a result of the increasing number of Civil War casualties. On July 17, 1862, Congress enacted legislation authorizing President Abraham Lincoln "to purchase cemetery grounds and cause them to be securely enclosed, to be used as a national cemetery for the soldiers who shall die in the service of the country."[43]

On September 11, 1861, the War Department, under "General Orders No. 75,"[44] made the Army's Quartermaster-General responsible for the burial of all officers and soldiers and for keeping a register of the burials. Before the 1862 legislation was enacted, soldiers were buried in family-selected private cemeteries, military post cemeteries, or at the sites of their deaths. In 1862, the first 14 national cemeteries were established.

After the Civil War ended in 1865, the Army Quartermaster Department began the Federal Reburial Program to "search for, recover, and identify the remains of all Union soldiers." Despite extensive efforts, many of the dead soldiers could not be located, and the identities of nearly half of those recovered and reburied were unknown. Approximately 300,000 Union soldiers were recovered by 1870 and buried in 73 national cemeteries, most of which were located in the southeastern United States near Civil War battlefields and campgrounds.

The National Cemetery Act of 1867, enacted by Congress on February 22, 1867, was the first major piece of legislation to provide funds and directives to national cemeteries.[45] A number of amendments to the National Cemetery Act of 1867 were passed in the 1870s. One enacted by Congress on March 3, 1873, expanded eligibility and permitted "the interment of honorably discharged Soldiers, Sailors, and Marines" in national cemeteries.[46] In response to this change, 47 new cemeteries were established; more durable marble headstones replaced the original wooden headstones; and Army Quartermaster-General Montgomery C. Meigs, with recommendations from landscape architect Frederick Law Olmsted, improved the aesthetics of the new cemeteries.

Near the end of the 19th century, former Union and Confederate soldiers began to reconcile their differences and seemed to develop a sense of unity. The feeling spread throughout the country and eventually to Washington, DC. As a result, 264 Confederate soldiers were "re-interred into a newly created 'Confederate section' at Arlington National Cemetery in 1901."

The 1930s proved to be a time of great change in operations for national cemeteries. Congress established the Veterans Administration (VA) in 1930 and made it responsible for the National Homes for Disabled Volunteer Soldiers (NHDVS), later referred to as the National Homes for Disabled Veterans, and the 21 cemeteries located on these properties. On July 10, 1933, Section 2 of Executive Order No. 6166 transferred 11 national cemeteries "from custody of the War Department and Army to the National Park Service (NPS) under the Department of the Interior (DOI)."[47] In 1934 eight World War I cemeteries established abroad were transferred to the custody of the American Battle Monuments Commission (ABMC).[48]

The next three decades were marked primarily by legislation that extended burial eligibility to certain categories of individuals who were not previously eligible to be buried in national cemeteries. In 1967, however, President Lyndon Johnson assigned the VA with the responsibility of conducting a survey of veteran and Army national cemetery programs. As a result of the report that the VA submitted on March 18, 1968, Congress passed the National Cemeteries Act of 1973 (P.L. 93-43), which authorized the transfer of 82 national cemeteries and the procurement of government headstones and markers from the Department of the Army to the Veterans Administration. The Army, however, maintained control and responsibility for Arlington National Cemetery in Arlington, VA, and The U.S. Soldiers' and Sailors' Home National Cemetery in Washington, DC.

When the official transfer took place on September 1, 1973, the VA elevated its 21 NHDVS cemeteries to the status of national cemeteries. Combined, the newly structured system consisted of 103 cemeteries. The 1973 act also permanently established the Advisory Committee on Cemeteries and Memorials. Under the VA, the National Cemetery System (NCS), in its first decade of operation, experienced the largest acreage expansion since the Civil War. Thirteen new national cemeteries were established during the 1970s and 1980s. In 1986, Congress passed the Veteran's Benefits Improvement and Health Care Authorization Act of 1986 (P.L. 99-576), which ordered the VA to identify the areas in the United States that were in the greatest need of veteran burial grounds.

On November 11, 1998, President Bill Clinton signed the Veterans Programs Enhancement Act of 1998 (P.L. 105-368). Section 403 of this law changed the name of the National Cemetery System to the National Cemetery Administration (NCA), and it elevated the position of Director of the National Cemetery System to Under Secretary for Memorial Affairs. In 1999, the Veterans Millennium Health Care and Benefits Act (P.L. 106-117) required the VA to study future burial needs and mandated the creation of six new national cemeteries in the areas where they were most needed. The National Cemetery Expansion Act of 2003 (P.L. 108-109), enacted on November 11, 2003, authorized the creation of the six new cemeteries.

Since the inception of national cemeteries in 1862, there have been more than 3 million burials in national cemeteries around the United States. Today, there are 131 national cemeteries, along with 33 soldier's lots and monument sites, under the jurisdiction of the VA.

Establishing National Cemeteries

The Secretary of VA has the authority to acquire land for national cemeteries "by purchase, gift (including donations from States or political subdivisions thereof), condemnation, transfer from other Federal agencies, exchange, or otherwise" at his discretion.[49] Although the Secretary has complete autonomy on where the cemeteries should be placed, the VA has a policy designed to place them in the areas where they are most needed.

Current VA policy establishes new national cemeteries in areas where there is no national or state veterans cemetery within a 75-mile radius, and where there is a population of at least 170,000 unserved veterans.[50] Building a new national cemetery is a six-step process: site selection; environmental assessment; land acquisition; master planning and design development; construction documents preparation; and construction award and completion.[51]

In addition to establishing national cemeteries, the VA assists in establishing state veterans cemeteries. The State Cemetery Grant Program established in 1978 provides burial funds for states, federally recognized tribal governments, or U.S. territories where national cemeteries do not meet veterans' burial needs. The VA can fund up to 100% of the development cost for the purpose of "establishing, expanding, or improving Veterans cemeteries."[52] Cemeteries established under the program must operate according to the rules, regulations, and guidelines of the National Cemetery Administration.[53]

Under the Veterans' Benefits Improvement and Health-Care Authorization Act of 1986 (P.L. 99-576), and more recently the Millennium Health Care and Benefits Act (P.L. 106-

117), Congress required the NCA to submit reports on the current and future need for national cemeteries. The reports are primarily logistical recommendations from the NCA on how best to reach their established goal of servicing 90% of veterans in need of burial services.[54]

To date, the VA has released four such reports. The 1987 and 1994 reports both identified 10 areas around the United States that were in the greatest need of veteran burial space and recommended against "NCS acquisition of state veterans' cemeteries … noting that the states were particularly useful in providing services in less populous areas."[55] The 1994 report also recommended continuing the expansion of existing cemeteries, stating that expansion is "a viable alternative to opening new cemeteries."[56] As a result of the reports, seven new cemeteries were established and a number of existing cemeteries were expanded.

The 2001 report submitted to Congress concluded that the establishment and first-year operation costs for a national cemetery range "between $16 million and $25 million."[57] The 2001 report also made the following major recommendations: "Continue to encourage grant program cemeteries; Continue to examine ways to expand the service life of existing cemeteries; Build new national cemeteries at or near the locations recommended … in combination with the previous options."[58]

According to the most recent 2008 report, "No location in the U.S. will meet the criteria for the establishment of a new national cemetery under the current service area standard (i.e., 75-miles, 170,000 veterans) until 2015."[59] At that time, the only community that would meet the qualifying population threshold of 170,000 would be the St. Louis, MO, metropolitan area because of the planned closing of Jefferson Barracks National Cemetery around 2017.[60] The report recommends retaining the 75-mile service area standard, but reducing the veteran population threshold from 170,000 to 110,000 to increase the number of unserved communities that could qualify for a new national cemetery. This change would allow two unserved communities to qualify for new national cemeteries: Charleston, WV, and Schuyler, NE.[61]

The Veterans' Benefits Act of 2010 (P.L. 111-275) required the Secretary to report, within one year, on the site selection, schedule for establishment, and required funding for establishment of new cemeteries in five areas: (1) in Southern California; (2) near Melbourne, FL and Daytona, FL; (3) near Omaha, NE; (4) near Buffalo, NY, and Rochester, NY; and (5) near Tallahassee, FL. The Secretary is required to report every two years afterword until the cemeteries are established.

LEGISLATION IN THE 111TH CONGRESS

A number of bills have been introduced in the 111th Congress that would affect nonmonetary and monetary burial benefits, and national cemeteries.

Nonmonetary Burial Benefits

The following legislation on nonmonetary burial benefits has been introduced in the 111th Congress:

H.R. 731—would prohibit any person classified as a tier III sex offender under the Sex Offender Registration and Notification Act from interment or memorialization in a cemetery under the National Cemetery Administration, Arlington National Cemetery, and certain state veterans cemeteries.

H.R. 2586—would prohibit the Secretary of Veterans Affairs (VA) from authorizing an honor guard to participate in the funeral of any veteran interred in a national cemetery under the control of the National Cemetery Administration unless the honor guard offers to the family the option of having it perform one of the 13-fold flag recitations.

H.R. 3949 (as passed by the House (H.Rept. 111-324))—would authorize interment in a national cemetery to parents of individuals who died in combat or from a combat-related training injury if those individuals are interred in a national cemetery and have no other eligible survivors. The benefit would be provided only if there is available gravesite space.

Monetary Burial Benefits

The following legislation on monetary burial benefits has been introduced in the 111th Congress:

H.R. 1037 (as amended and passed in the Senate)—would increase from $300 to $745 the VA payment for (1) burial and funeral expenses of a veteran who dies in a VA hospital, nursing home, or domiciliary care facility; and (2) a plot allowance for a veteran eligible for burial in a national cemetery who is not buried in a national cemetery. The bill also would provide for an annual adjustment of these amounts based on increases in the Consumer Price Index (CPI).

H.R. 2594—would provide a $300 plot allowance to a state for the interment in state cemeteries of spouses and children of certain veterans who are buried in state cemeteries.

H.R. 4044—would make the plot allowance available to any veteran of war and restore the pre-1990 headstone allowance.

H.R. 4045—would increase the level of the monetary annual allowances and provide for annual inflation adjustment (equal to the Social Security cost-of-living adjustment).

H.R. 6042—would permit the Secretary of VA under certain circumstances to pay the funeral expenses of certain homeless veterans who did not serve during a period of war.

S. 728—would provide, to the extent funds are available, a $900 supplemental payment for burial and funeral expenses for non-service-connected deaths and $2,000 for service-connected deaths. The bill also would provide for an annual increase in the amounts based on the CPI.

National Cemeteries

The following legislation on national cemeteries has been introduced in the 111th Congress:

H.R. 174 and S. 691—would direct VA to establish a new national cemetery for veterans in El Paso County, CO.

H.R. 217—would direct VA to acquire, subject to available appropriations, a specified parcel of land in Beaufort, SC, to be used for expansion of the Beaufort National Cemetery. The bill also would grant the VA the authority to accept donations of land.

H.R. 1114—would direct VA to establish a process for determining whether a geographic area is sufficiently served by the national cemeteries located in that area, taking into account, among other things, (1) the number of veterans living in the area; and (2) the average distance a resident of the area must travel to reach the nearest national cemetery. In the case of an area with insufficient land to establish a cemetery, the VA must consider alternatives such as establishing a mausoleum.

H.R. 1163 and S. 746—would direct VA to establish a national cemetery in Sarpy County, NE.

H.R. 2642—would direct VA to cooperate with veteran service organizations to assist entities in possession of unclaimed or abandoned human remains to determine if any such remains are the remains of veterans or other individuals eligible for burial in a national cemetery. The bill would require VA, upon a positive determination with respect to any such remains, to provide for and cover the cost of the burial and funeral expenses if the Secretary determines that (1) there is no next of kin or other person claiming the remains; and (2) there are no other sufficient resources to cover such expenses. The bill also would direct the Secretary to establish a publicly accessible national database of the names of any veterans or other individuals identified.

H.R. 3544—would direct VA to give priority to a location where at least 110,000 veterans reside within a 75-mile radius. It also would require the Secretary, in conducting an annual performance measure of the percentage of veterans served by a cemetery, to (1) use census tracts, rather than counties, to test and identify potential cemetery locations and to determine the percentage of veterans served; (2) use methods to avoid the double counting of veterans in overlapping service areas; and (3) count veterans who reside in counties bisected by a service area using a proportional overlay method.

H.R. 5879—would expand eligibility for interment in national cemeteries to individuals who supported the United States in Laos during the Vietnam War era.

Appendix A. Legislative History of Monetary Burial Benefits (Funeral, Burial, and Plot Allowances)

The earliest reference to a federal monetary burial allowance for veterans was during World War I. Changes that were made to the burial allowance for veterans between 1917 and 2001 are as follows:

1917: War Risk Insurance Act Amendment (P.L. 65-90)

Provided a maximum payment of $100 for a veteran's burial expenses and the return of the veteran's remains to his home if the death occurred before discharge or resignation from military service.

1924: World War Veterans' Act, 1924 (P.L. 68-242)

Established service-connected and non-service-connected burial allowances of $100.

1933: P.L. 73-2

Increased both service-connected and non-service-connected burial allowances to $107.

1936: P.L. 74-844

Provided that the burial allowance would not be denied based on the deceased veteran's net assets at the time of death. This law further established a one-year limit after burial for filing a claim for the allowance; required the Veterans Administration (VA) to notify the claimant of any information required to complete the claim; and stipulated that the allowance would not be granted if the evidence was not provided within one year of the date of the request.

1957: Veterans Benefits Act of 1957 (P.L. 85-56)

Provided a burial allowance of $150 to cover burial and funeral expenses, preparation of the body, and transportation to the place of burial for a deceased veteran of any war who had been discharged from active military service due to disability or was receiving disability compensation. The burial allowance was not to be denied based on the veteran's net assets at the time of death. The allowance would be reduced by any contributions paid by a government agency, the deceased veteran's employer, or a burial association, and the balance of the burial allowance (up to the $150) would be paid to the claimant.

1958: P.L. 85-674

Increased the burial allowance to $250.

1958: P.L. 85-857

Mandated VA to pay the $250 burial allowance for a veteran who died in a VA facility if the veteran had been properly admitted for hospital or domiciliary care. The VA was permitted to enter into contracts to provide the burial and funeral services for veterans who died in VA facilities. P.L. 85-857 also mandated the VA to pay for transporting the bodies of veterans who died in VA facilities to the place of burial; and clarified that the $250 burial allowance was not to be paid for deaths prior to August 19, 1958. P.L. 85-857 also extended the filing period for reimbursement claims to two years after the burial of the veteran.

1964: P.L. 88-359

Eliminated the offset against the VA burial allowances for amounts paid by burial associations.

1966: P.L. 89-360

Extended the $250 burial allowance to peacetime veterans who died because of service-connected disabilities but had not applied for disability compensation.

1973: National Cemeteries Act of 1973 (P.L. 93-43)

Provided a plot or interment allowance of $150 for veterans who were not buried in national cemeteries. This allowance was applied to the difference between the total plot or interment expenses and the amount paid by a state, a state agency or subdivision, or the deceased veteran's employer. P.L. 93-43 also required the VA to provide headstones or markers for unmarked graves of veterans buried in national or military post/base cemeteries; certain individuals eligible for burial in national cemeteries, but not buried in national cemeteries; and soldiers of the Union and Confederate Armies of the Civil War. The VA also was mandated to provide headstones or markers, when requested, for veterans whose remains had not been recovered or were buried at sea for placement by the applicants. P.L. 93-43 also provided that the survivors of veterans who died due to service-connected disabilities may request that the VA pay burial and funeral expenses at the amount authorized for the death of a federal employee due to an injury incurred in the performance of duty ($800) instead of the standard VA burial and plot allowances.

1978: Veterans' Housing Benefits Improvement Act of 1978 (P.L. 95-476)

Extended the $150 plot allowance to states (or their political subdivisions) for the burial of veterans eligible for burial in national cemeteries in state veterans cemeteries. If the veterans are not buried in cemeteries (or portions of cemeteries) that are solely for the interment of persons eligible for burial in national cemeteries, the plot allowance is limited to those total costs not paid by the states (or their political subdivisions) or the veterans' employers.

1978: Veterans Disability Compensation and Survivors' Benefits Act of 1978 (P.L. 95-479)

Increased the burial allowance to $300. P.L. 95-479 also limited the burial and funeral expenses paid for a veteran who died of a service-connected disability to $1,100.

1981: Omnibus Budget Reconciliation Act of 1981 (P.L. 97-35)

Limited payment of the burial allowance to the cases of veterans who were eligible to receive pensions or disability compensation.

1982: Veterans' Compensation, Education, and Employment Amendments of 1982 (P.L. 97-306)

Provided that the VA administrator may pay the burial allowance to states (or their political subdivisions) that are holding the bodies of eligible indigent deceased veterans whose remains are unclaimed and for whom there are insufficient resources to cover burial and funeral expenses. P.L. 97-306 also provided that the burial allowance would be paid for veterans who died in VA-contracted nursing homes.

1988: Veterans' Benefits and Services Act of 1988 (P.L. 100-322)

Increased the burial allowance for veterans who died from service-connected disabilities to $1,500.

1996: Veterans' Benefits Improvements Act of 1996 (P.L. 104-275)

Provided that a $300 burial allowance would be paid for veterans who died in state nursing homes.

2000: Veterans Benefits and Health Care Improvement Act of 2000 (P.L. 106-419)

Extended the plot and interment allowance for burial in state veterans' cemeteries to members, or former members, of Armed Forces reserve components not otherwise eligible for burial in national cemeteries. This law also extended eligibility for interment in national cemeteries to certain Filipino veterans of World War II.

2001: Veterans Education and Benefits Expansion Act of 2001 (P.L. 107-103)

Increased the plot allowance to $300 and the burial and funeral allowance for veterans who died due to service-connected disabilities to $2,000.

2010: Veterans' Benefits Act of 2010 (P.L. 111-275)

Increased plot allowance to $700 effective October 1, 2011, and provided for an inflation adjustment beginning in FY2013.

APPENDIX B. LEGISLATIVE HISTORY OF NATIONAL CEMETERIES

The earliest reference to the national cemetery program is found in General Orders No. 75 (1861). Subsequent major changes that were made to the national cemetery program are as follows:[62]

1861: General Orders No. 75

Made Quartermaster responsible for the burial of (Union) officers and soldiers and for keeping a register of all burials. Also stipulated that a headstone was to be placed at the head of each grave.

1867: National Cemetery Act (Chapter 61 of the Acts of the 39th Congress)

Provided funds and set guidelines for the establishment and protection of national cemeteries.

1872: Chapter 173 of the Acts of the 42nd Congress

Authorized the Secretary of War to appoint "meritorious and trustworthy" soldiers as superintendents of national cemeteries.

1872: Chapter 257 of the Acts of the 42nd Congress

Amended the National Cemetery Act to allow all honorably discharged soldiers and sailors who were destitute to be buried in national cemeteries.

1873: Chapter 276 of the Acts of the 42nd Congress

Allowed all honorably discharged soldiers, sailors, and marines who served in the Civil War in the regular or volunteer forces to be buried in national cemeteries at no cost.

1906: P.L. 59-38

Provided for the appropriate marking of the graves of Confederate soldiers and sailors who died in northern prisons and military hospitals and were buried near those prisons and hospitals.

1920: P.L. 66-175

Expanded eligibility for burial in national cemeteries to U.S. citizens "who served in the Army or Navy of any government at war with Germany or Austria during the World War" and who died during service or after being honorably discharged.

1923: P.L. 67-534

Established the American Battle Monuments Commission to erect suitable memorials commemorating the service of American soldiers in Europe.

1930: P.L. 71-536

Established the Veterans Administration (VA) and made it responsible for the National Homes for Disabled Volunteer Soldiers (NHDVS) and the 21 cemeteries located on those properties.

1933: Executive Order No. 6166

Transferred 11 national cemeteries from the custody of the War Department and the Army to the National Park Service under the Department of the Interior.

1948: P.L. 80-526

Expanded eligibility for burial in a national cemetery to the eligible survivors of veterans.

1959: P.L. 86-260

Expanded eligibility for burial in national cemeteries to Army or Air National Guard and Reserves and to Reserve Officer Training Corps (ROTC) members if they were doing exercises or were on active duty at the time of death.

1973: National Cemetery Act of 1973 (P.L. 93-43)

Transferred custody of national cemeteries from the Army to VA's newly established National Cemetery System. VA cemeteries were elevated to national cemetery status. The Army retained control of Arlington National Cemetery and the cemetery at the U.S. Soldiers' and Airmen's Home. The NCS was given responsibility for veterans' headstones and markers. This law distinguished between service-connected and non-service-connected deaths for allowances. It added benefit of transportation of remains under certain circumstances.

1978: Veterans' Housing Benefits Act of 1978 (P.L. 95-476)

Authorized the VA to pay a $150 burial allowance to states for the burial of veterans eligible to be buried in national cemeteries in state veterans' cemeteries. Authorized a program of grant assistance to states to establish, expand, and improve state veterans' cemeteries.

1986: Veterans' Benefits Improvement and Health-Care Authorization Act of 1986 (P.L. 99-576)

Mandated the VA to conduct studies to identify the 10 geographic areas within the United States with the greatest need for additional veterans' burial space.

1998: Veterans Programs Enhancement Act of 1998 (P.L. 105-368)

Redesignated the National Cemetery System as the National Cemetery Administration, and designated the position of Director of the National Cemetery System as the Under Secretary for Memorial Affairs. Also extended eligibility for burial in a national cemetery to qualified merchant mariners.

1999: Veterans Millennium Health Care and Benefits Act (P.L. 106-117)

Directed the VA Secretary to contract with one or more qualified organizations to conduct independent studies for improvements to veterans' burial benefits and for improvements to veterans' cemeteries. Mandated the Secretary to establish national cemeteries in the six U.S. areas where they are most needed.

2003: National Cemetery Expansion Act of 2003 (P.L. 108-109)

Authorized the establishment of six new national cemeteries in the following areas: Birmingham, AL; Bakersfield, CA; Jacksonville, FL; Sarasota County, FL; southeastern Pennsylvania; and Greenville/Columbia, SC.

2003: Veterans Benefits Act of 2003 (P.L. 108-183)

Expanded eligibility for burial in a national cemetery to remarried surviving spouses of deceased veterans. Permanently authorized the state veterans' cemeteries grant program under the VA.

2010: Veterans' Benefits Act of 2010 (P.L. 111-275)

Expanded eligibility for burial in a national cemetery to parents of certain interred veterans. Required a new study for establishing cemeteries in five designated areas.

End Notes

[1] For a detailed description of disability compensation and pension programs, see CRS Report RL34626, *Veterans' Benefits: Benefits Available for Disabled Veterans*, by Christine Scott and Carol D. Davis; CRS Report RL33323, *Veterans Affairs: Benefits for Service-Connected Disabilities*, by Douglas Reid Weimer; and CRS Report RS22804, *Veterans' Benefits: Pension Benefit Programs*, by Christine Scott and Carol D. Davis.

[2] For a discussion of education benefits, see CRS Report R40723, *Educational Assistance Programs Administered by the U.S. Department of Veterans Affairs*, by Cassandria Dortch.

[3] For details on VA's vocational rehabilitation and employment program, see CRS Report RL34627, *Veterans' Benefits: The Vocational Rehabilitation and Employment Program*, by Christine Scott and Carol D. Davis.

[4] For detailed information on homeless veterans programs, see CRS Report RL34024, *Veterans and Homelessness*, by Libby Perl.

[5] For details on the home loan guarantee program, see CRS Report RS20533, *VA-Home Loan Guaranty Program: An Overview*, by Bruce E. Foote.

[6] Established by the National Cemeteries Act of 1973 (P.L. 93-43).

[7] Next of kin—recognized in order: surviving spouse; children, according to age; parents, including adoptive, stepparents, and foster parents; brothers or sisters, including half or step brothers and sisters; grandparents; grandchildren; uncles or aunts; nephews or nieces; cousins; and/or other lineal descendent. For more information, see 38 C.F.R. § 38.633.

[8] The term "service-connected" refers to deaths that occurred while on active duty or due to a condition incurred in or aggravated by active duty. The term "non-service-connected" refers to deaths that did not occur while on active duty or due to a condition that was not incurred in or aggravated by active duty.

[9] The term "soldier's lots" refers to the section of a public or private cemetery reserved for the interment of soldiers. These sections are under the purview of the nearest national cemetery.

[10] 38 C.F.R. § 38.620.

[11] For detailed information on other than dishonorable discharges, see CRS Report RL33113, *Veterans Affairs: Basic Eligibility for Disability Benefit Programs*, by Douglas Reid Weimer.

[12] The veteran does not have to be deceased for the spouse or dependents to receive this benefit.

[13] Hostile casualty is defined as a member of the Armed Forces who dies as the result of hostile action with the enemy, while in combat, while traveling to or from combat if death was related to hostile action, while hospitalized or undergoing treatment for injuries incurred during combat, or was killed mistakenly or accidentally by friendly fire directed at or thought to be directed at a hostile force. It does not include persons

who die due to elements, self-inflicted wounds, combat fatigue, or by friendly fire while in an absent-without-leave, deserter, or dropped-from-rolls status, or voluntarily absent from a place of duty.

[14] Effective for deaths of a parent on or after October 7, 2010.

[15] 38 U.S.C. § 2402(6).

[16] For more information on national cemetery burial ineligibility, see VA website's "Eligibility" page at http://www.cem.va.gov/bbene/eligible.asp.

[17] 38 U.S.C. § 2411.

[18] Prior to the Omnibus Budget Reconciliation Act of 1990 (P.L. 101-508), the VA provided headstone allowances for veterans eligible to be buried in a national cemetery, who were buried in a private cemetery. For more information, see P.L. 101-508, Sections 8041-8042.

[19] For more information, see 38 C.F.R. § 30.632.

[20] For more information, see the "Government-Furnished Headstones and Markers" page on the VA website at http://www.cem.va.gov/pdf/hm.pdf.

[21] See http://www4.va.gov/vaforms/va/pdf/VA40-1330.pdf.

[22] 38 C.F.R. § 38.632.

[23] The list of approved emblems of belief can be viewed at http://www.cem.va.gov/hm/hmemb.asp.

[24] For more information, see the "Presidential Memorial Certificates" page on the VA website at http://www.cem.va.gov/pdf/pmc.pdf.

[25] See http://www4.va.gov/vaforms/va/pdf/VA40-0247.pdf.

[26] Department of Veterans Affairs, *Evaluation of the VA Burial Benefits Program: Final Report,* August 2008, pp. 99-126, http://www1.va.gov/op3/docs/ProgramEvaluations/Final_Burial_Report_8-26-08.pdf.

[27] Ibid., pp. 100, 126.

[28] Avenue of Flags is a traditional name used to describe a large display of American flags.

[29] For more information, see the "Burial Flags" page on the VA website at http://www.cem.va.gov/pdf/flags.pdf.

[30] See http://www.vba.va.gov/pubs/forms/VBA-21-2008-ARE.pdf.

[31] For the Legislative History of Monetary Burial Benefits see **Appendix A**.

[32] For more information, see the "Burial and Plot-Interment Allowances" page on the VA website at http://www.cem.va.gov/bbene/benvba.asp.

[33] 38 U.S.C. § 2302.

[34] State includes any political subdivision or agency of a state.

[35] 38 U.S.C. § 2302.

[36] 38 U.S.C. § 2402.

[37] 38 U.S.C. § 2307.

[38] Department of Veterans Affairs, *Evaluation of the VA Burial Benefits Program: Final Report*, August 2008, p. 153, http://www1.va.gov/op3/docs/ProgramEvaluations/Final_Burial_Report_8-26-08.pdf.

[39] Ibid., pp. 152-162.

[40] Ibid., p. 161.

[41] Ibid., pp. 161-162.

[42] More detailed history is available on the VA website on the "History and Development of the National Cemetery Administration" page at http://www.cem.va.gov/pdf/history.pdf. For the Legislative History of National Cemeteries see **Appendix B**.

[43] 12 Stat. 596, Ch. 200 (1862).

[44] The text is available on the National Park Service Website at http://www.nps.gov/history/Nr/twhp/wwwlps/lessons/ 115dayton/115facts3.htm.

[45] 14 Stat. 399, Ch. 39 (1867).

[46] 17 Stat. 605, Ch. 276 (1873).

[47] The text of Executive Order No. 6166 is available on the National Archives and Records Administration Website at http://www.archives.gov/federal-register/codification/executive-order/06166.html.

[48] For more information on the American Battle Monuments Commission (ABMC), see the ABMC website at http://www.abmc.gov/commission/index.php.

[49] 38 U.S.C. § 2406.

[50] Unserved veterans are those veterans without the option of a national or state cemetery within 75 miles.

[51] For more information, see the VA website's "National Cemetery Development" page at http://www.cem.va.gov/pdf/ newcemdev.pdf.

[52] For more information, see the VA website's "State Cemetery Grants Program – General Information" page at http://www.cem.va.gov/scg/scgpinfo.asp.

[53] Ibid.

[54] Logistics Management Institute, Veterans Millennium Health Care and Benefits Act of 1999 Study on Improvements to Veterans Cemeteries, Volume 1: Future Burial Needs, December 2001, pp. 1-3.

[55] Ibid.

[56] Ibid., pp. 1-3.

[57] Ibid., pp. 3-12.

[58] Ibid., pp. 3-12.

[59] Department of Veterans Affairs, *Evaluation of the VA Burial Benefits Program: Final Report*, August 2008, p. 73, http://www1.va.gov/op3/docs/ProgramEvaluations/Final_Burial_Report_8-26-08.pdf.

[60] Ibid., p. 165.

[61] Ibid., p. 74 (PDF p. 101).

[62] Department of Veterans Affairs, *Evaluation of the VA Burial Benefits Program: Final Report*, August 2008, pp. 15-20 (PDF), http://www1.va.gov/op3/docs/ProgramEvaluations/Final_Burial_Report_8-26-08.pdf.

CHAPTER SOURCES

The following chapters have been previously published:

Chapter 1 – This is an edited, excerpted and augmented edition of a United States Congressional Research Service publication, Report Order Code R40757, dated October 18, 2010.

Chapter 2 – This is an edited, excerpted and augmented edition of a United States Congressional Research Service publication, Report Order Code RS22483, dated February 18, 2010.

Chapter 3 – This is an edited, excerpted and augmented edition of a United States Congressional Research Service publication, Report Order Code RL33323, dated June 16, 2010.

Chapter 4 – This is an edited, excerpted and augmented edition of a United States Congressional Research Service publication, Report Order Code RL34626, dated October 18, 2010.

Chapter 5 – This is an edited, excerpted and augmented edition of a United States Congressional Research Service publication, Report Order Code R41065, dated February 3, 2010.

Chapter 6 – This is an edited, excerpted and augmented edition of a United States Congressional Research Service publication, Report Order Code RL34370, dated September 22, 2010.

Chapter 7 – This is an edited, excerpted and augmented edition of a United States Congressional Research Service publication, Report Order Code R41435, dated October 18, 2010.

Chapter 8 – This is an edited, excerpted and augmented edition of a United States Congressional Research Service publication, Report Order Code RS22666, dated April 9, 2010.

Chapter 9 – This is an edited, excerpted and augmented edition of a United States Congressional Research Service publication, Report Order Code RL34627, dated October 18, 2010.

Chapter 10 – This is an edited, excerpted and augmented edition of a United States Congressional Research Service publication, Report Order Code R40273, dated February 1, 2010.

Chapter 11 - This is an edited, excerpted and augmented edition of a United States Congressional Research Service publication, Report Order Code RSS2804, dated October 18, 2010.

Chapter 12 - This is an edited, excerpted and augmented edition of a United States Congressional Research Service publication, Report Order Code R41386, dated October 18, 2010.

INDEX

E

F

J

K

L

M

N

O

P

Q